This book will have you exp[eriencing]
sadness, and everything in b[etween].
Down syndrome will be a[ware]
heartwarming story—and it is a blueprint for how we should all
fight for our children's rights.
    —Dennis Dykes, director, Canadian Down Syndrome Society

An affectionate memoir . . . poignant . . . humorous . . . deeply
affecting.   *—Sidney Allinson, Victoria Times Colonist newspaper*

A gentle, yet powerful story of the profound love between a
mother and her child. An interesting read for every parent and
every educator. This book is a strong reminder that children
learn from their peers, and that *all* children have many gifts to
share.   *—Sue Johnston, educator*

I laughed at some parts, cried at others, felt anxious, distressed,
happy, hopeful—it did exactly what a book needs to do—give
the reader feelings. A sensitively written work full of love and
insight. A book as special as the child whose story it tells.
    —Ann Alma, author of bestselling novel, "Summer of Changes"

A beautiful tribute which also acknowledges the cause—and
positive effect—of foster parenting.
    —Tracey Morrissey, medical foster parent for the State of Missouri

The pain and suffering, both of Jade and of those who loved her,
were enormous. But outweighing that tremendously, joyfully
bursting forth, is the incredible richness of her life and the many,
many blessings that were delivered through this little girl.
        —Marsha Henderson, parent

As a healthcare professional, I've gained greater insight into the
triumphs and tribulations of a critically ill child. Deeply moving
with a good dose of humour. Jade is a real scene-stealer, who
inevitably stole my heart!   *—Maureen Garland, RN*

Natural Harmony
Jade's Story

Gail Albrechtson

Printed in Victoria, Canada

Edited by Patricia Anderson, PhD

Cover Art by Sheena Lott

National Library of Canada Cataloguing in Publication

Albrechtson, Gail
    Natural harmony : Jade's story / Gail Albrechtson.
ISBN 1-4120-0392-X
    1. Albrechtson, Gail. 2. Down syndrome--Biography.
    3. Albrechtson family.

RJ506.D68A43 2003   362.1'96858842'0092   C2003-902861-5

TRAFFORD

This book was published *on-demand* in cooperation with Trafford Publishing.
On-demand publishing is a unique process and service of making a book available for retail sale to the public taking advantage of on-demand manufacturing and Internet marketing.
On-demand publishing includes promotions, retail sales, manufacturing, order fulfilment, accounting and collecting royalties on behalf of the author.

Suite 6E, 2333 Government St., Victoria, B.C. V8T 4P4, CANADA
Phone   250-383-6864   Toll-free   1-888-232-4444 (Canada & US)
Fax   250-383-6804   E-mail   sales@trafford.com
Web site   www.trafford.com   TRAFFORD PUBLISHING IS A DIVISION OF TRAFFORD HOLDINGS LTD.
Trafford Catalogue #03-0761   www.trafford.com/robots/03-0761.html

10   9   8   7   6   5   4   3

In loving memory of Jade

(July 1, 1979 – January 12, 1986)

for

Jim and Joan Pearson

PROLOGUE

It was a beautiful sunny morning, around eleven thirty, when I met Jade at the schoolyard. I was so happy to be picking up my daughter from kindergarten—thrilled with the whole concept that she was even attending school, let alone a regular school with regular kids.

I scanned the large groups of children leaving the building. Anticipating Jade's happy face, I looked around but couldn't see Jade in any group. Then I spotted her by the chain-link fence. Looking quite dejected, she just stood there. There was no cheerful greeting, no smile, no kisses, no hugs—nothing.

My God, I thought, maybe the special education teachers were right. Maybe the social workers, along with all the other professionals, were right. Maybe Jade doesn't fit in with normal children. Maybe she's been ridiculed, rejected, and left to cry in some corner of the classroom, just like they said she would. Maybe all of my efforts toward her successful integration into a normal school have indeed proven to be a failure, just as the experts had predicted.

Wanting to walk home with her and talk about her morning's experience, I took Jade's hand, but she pulled hers away and held onto the metal fence. Finally she looked up, and her eyes met mine.

"No papo," she said in a quivering voice, "Miss Kine gimme no papo." Accusingly, Jade looked over toward the teacher, who was speaking with another parent. "I wan one," she said, "I wanna papo!"

I had a private chat with Miss Klein. She explained that

the children who knew their address and telephone number were awarded a sheet of paper, on which was a picture of a house and a written acknowledgement that the child had indeed learned his or her own contact information.

"I can't believe how hurt Jade is over this," she said, "but I can't very well give an award sheet to her when half the class couldn't give their address either. For safety reasons, it's important that the children know this information. Each child has been reassured that once he or she has learned it, they will then receive an award sheet."

As we walked home, I tried to explain to my deeply disappointed little girl that many of the students didn't receive a paper— it wasn't just her. Jade hadn't said a word all the while. We no sooner got through the front door, when she let it all out. I picked her up and she clung to me, her arms tight around my neck and her legs wrapped around my waist. She sobbed into my neck. I was so annoyed with myself for not having taught Jade this vital information. That piece of paper meant so much to her, and it hurt me to think how disappointed she felt because she "hadn't got it."

That afternoon, I was determined to teach Jade what she needed to know. We went out for a walk, observing and pointing out all the little number signs that indicated an address. We walked to the corner, and I pointed out the street sign. We made up songs: "Where do you live? I live at 319A Westminister Avenue." By the end of that afternoon, Jade knew her address, but as for her phone number—that was a tough one and would probably require an additional day's practice.

Two days later, while I prepared lunch, a friend of mine met Jade at school. She later mentioned that Jade hadn't said a word all the way home, yet had a mischievous grin on her face. When Jade walked in the front door, she headed straight for the kitchen to see me. With a beaming smile on her face, she plunked her backpack onto the table, then pulled something out.

"*I got it!*" She waved it in the air. "*I gotta papo!*"

It was moments like this that made me want to scream

out with joy.

This is the story of my late daughter, Jade, and the six and a half years that she so lovingly enriched my life. It is a story that has been at the back of my mind for the past seventeen years, and now, finally, I'm going to fulfill a longstanding desire to preserve Jade's memory by sharing some anecdotes, her keen sense of humour, and all the simple, loving ways in which she managed to touch people's hearts.

Those six and a half years, when I think about them now, seem to have disappeared in a flash. They were the years that changed my life, a time when I no longer pondered "the meaning of life," for I had learned it the moment I first looked into my daughter's eyes. During her brief time with me, Jade became my everything—my whole life, my whole heart, and my whole spirit.

CHAPTER ONE

As I lay in bed one night I thought there must be something very religious about being pregnant, because I could not fall asleep without first saying a few prayers for the baby and reassuring him or her of the love that awaited.

I looked forward to retiring at night because it was the only time I had to really think. I found myself getting lonelier by the day, as I anticipated the birth more and more.

One evening while out walking my two dogs, a Chihuahua mix and a Doberman pinscher, I began to have contractions. I still had about a mile to walk home, but by stopping to rest every ten minutes or so, I finally made it back.

I informed my then husband Martin about the contractions, and by 11 P.M. I was checked into Montreal General Hospital. But the dilation was only at one centimetre, and the doctor advised me to return home until the contractions became more severe.

I tried to sleep but couldn't. Anxious and worried, I somehow thought that if I fell asleep I'd miss out on the whole thing. The following morning, back in the hospital, I was told the dilation had only increased by one centimetre. I returned to the hospital around four o'clock in the afternoon. All the while we were driving there, I couldn't believe that I was finally going to meet my baby within the next few hours or so. I started to think of names again: Mathew, James, Stephen, and other favourite masculine names. Because I terribly missed my four-year-old nephew, who had moved out of town with his divorced dad, I'd been wanting a boy so badly that it almost didn't occur to me that

1

it might, just might, be a girl.

In the Case Room I became a statistic on a big chalkboard—just a last name and a dilation number. By this time a doctor had determined the dilation to be at four centimetres. When she completed the examination, I started to sob uncontrollably.

Concerned, the doctor turned to me and said, "I realize that you are not very comfortable, but what's making you so upset? Has something happened? It isn't normal to be so depressed at a time like this. You are going to have a baby; you should be happy."

I had a whole slew of reasons for my unhappiness but wasn't about to divulge any of them to a stranger, sympathetic or not.

The doctor assigned me a private room on the maternity ward and prescribed some medication to help me sleep. But I still couldn't sleep, as the labour pains were now extremely severe.

Hours later, I could no longer stand the pain and vowed that the next child, should there be a next, would be adopted. I kept calling for a nurse, or somebody, anybody, to come and help me. A resident female doctor entered the room, examined me, and said, "It won't be much longer now."

The doctor mentioned that the exceptionally prolonged labour was probably due to my tired, tense state. She then asked if I could walk to the delivery room. *Walk?* I couldn't believe it—this doctor must have never had labour pains! She held my arm as I staggered down the corridor. Hoping to spot a wheelchair, I scanned the green, sterile aisle. I thought the baby was going to drop out, right then and there.

A half hour later, the blessed event finally came about. And it really is true that giving birth is the most beautiful and gratifying experience. As soon as the baby emerged, I instantly forgot all pain and discomfort.

A *girl*. For a second, I thought the doctor should double-check. I was ecstatic. As the nurses were washing the baby and preparing her for our first meeting, I couldn't stop laughing. When they placed her in my arms I couldn't believe that she was

2

finally here. So beautiful. *She*—I was still getting used to the term *she* —was staring up at me as if to say, "What's going on?"

Alone with this beautiful infant, I sensed that there was something extraordinarily special about her. She was just so, so precious. A name then came to mind: "Jade," as in the precious gem.

I don't think I had my baby for five minutes when she was whisked from my arms and taken away to the nursery. I was brought to my room and, with a feeling of gratitude, instantly fell asleep.

I awakened about six hours later, and practically felt like pinching myself to make sure that this great feeling was for real. I leaped out of bed and proceeded down the corridor to the shower room. With the warm water spraying over my body, I felt as though I was being reborn, as though happiness had finally arrived after a long, long wait.

Famished, I returned to my room and ate some cold, mushy oatmeal and soggy toast. While seated on the bedside chair, I noticed several nurses with babies in their arms, strolling down the hallway en route to anxious mothers' arms. I was trying to imagine how happy I was going to be in the next few minutes. I waited and waited. Where's mine, I wondered?

Worried, I decided to walk over to the nursery to see Jade. She wasn't there. I asked the first nurse in sight, "Where's my baby? Why hasn't she been brought to me?" A calm young nurse replied, "Oh well, she must be in the Special Care Nursery." "Must be?" I asked. "You mean you don't know?"

After being directed, I literally ran to the Special Care Nursery where I asked a nurse why Jade was placed in this particular nursery. I was informed that because she was just a little over five pounds, having lost some weight after birth, she needed the specialized care provided to premature babies.

And there she was—so beautiful, so tiny. She was sleeping in an incubator, although her little body was twitching due to what appeared to be hiccups. I put my hands through the sockets of the incubator to touch her soft, warm skin.

One of the nurses then told me that they were waiting for

the pediatrician to complete her rounds, and that Jade would be brought to me shortly. Feeling much more at ease, I returned to my room and fell asleep.

A little while later, the pediatrician, Dr. O'Reilly, entered my room. With a concerned look on her face, she told me that she suspected certain anomalies in my baby. My heart sank.

She began, "Your baby seems to be lethargic. She has slanted eyes, smaller hands, and a smaller head than normal, but this is not to say that your baby is not normal. She may very well be normal, but a genetic specialist has been summoned in to run some tests."

I couldn't say a word. I helplessly watched the doctor's face, tears burning my eyes, as I waited for her to say, "No, I'm sorry, there's been a mistake." But she didn't.

I sat there for the longest time, waiting for the doctor's return. I knew there had to be a mistake and that she would come back with a cheerier, if embarrassed, look upon her face, to tell me about the error. Amazingly, I fell asleep. I hoped and prayed that I would wake up to find that everything, except for Jade, was just a terrible dream.

Within the next hour or so, the genetic specialist had arrived, and again I heard that my baby was suspected of having certain anomalies. Whatever my child had—no medical term would be given just yet—might affect various organs of the body, but "not to worry, because it's not my fault and there's nothing I can do."

Soon after the specialist had left, Martin arrived. I told him of the brief consultation that had just taken place. I cried for him, I cried for myself, and most of all, I cried for our baby.

We went into the nursery to see Jade. Such a beautiful infant! We wondered how anyone could possibly suspect that there were any abnormalities in someone who was just so perfect. We couldn't stop admiring her; it was an exhilarating moment. Here I was, holding our very own baby—not a doll, but a real live, squirming, lovable baby. Her eyes were deep blue, bright, and intense.

I tried but failed to breast-feed, for Jade would not

respond. Her sleep was more important, I guessed. The nurses were tending to her feeding just then, at least until she showed signs of being ready to drink on her own. After changing her diaper, cuddling, and touching her, I placed her back into the incubator. I assured her of our love and, at that very moment, was determined that everything was going to be all right.

That evening, with hopes of feeding my baby, I went into the nursery and was shocked to discover what appeared to be a violent type of feeding procedure. One of the special care nurses was holding Jade on her lap and inserting a straw-like tube down her tiny throat. Jade was gagging. Before I could say anything, the nurse explained the purpose of the particular feeding method: "By doing it this way we are certain that the milk is going directly into the baby's stomach."

At the time, not fully appreciating the efforts and responsibilities of the nurses, I cried, "You didn't even give me a chance! My breasts are sore and you didn't even give me a chance to at least try to feed my baby!"

I then began to realize that the nurses really were very kind, and I reminded myself how gentle and loving they are with the babies. It was then they suggested that I check the chart for feeding times, which would have to be followed exactly.

I requested that nobody visit me that night. I didn't think I could even make eye contact with anybody, at least not without falling apart. The turn of events had just been too much.

It was a long holiday weekend, and the wait for Jade's prognosis, whatever it might be, was going to be delayed. The worry was becoming so intense that I just wanted to scream at somebody—anybody. I didn't want our lives to be put on hold any longer.

Later that night in the nursery, Jade was sound asleep; I was told that she had just been fed a few minutes earlier. "Why didn't someone come to get me?" I asked. "I've been lying in bed, forcing myself to stay awake in order not to miss the next feeding!" Apparently, Jade had awakened earlier than expected, and feeding her was the practical thing to do at the time.

I returned to my room, cried in frustration, then fell

asleep.

After awaking the next morning with a throbbing headache, I showered, ate what they called breakfast, then went to the nursery at 7:30 A.M. It was such a relief when Jade finally drank some of my breast milk. She seemed more alert now, her eyes taking in every detail of my hands and face and, whenever there was a noise in the room, she tried to focus her attention on it. Finally, I truly felt like I was Jade's mother. I washed and changed her, and afterward couldn't help but marvel at this beautiful little being as she rested in my arms.

An hour had gone by, Jade still in my arms, when a nurse advised me that the baby needed her sleep and should be returned to her crib. So much for feeling like Jade's mother!

Throughout the day I was back and forth to the nursery. Except for a couple of successful attempts at breast-feeding, Jade wouldn't respond, instead falling asleep in my arms. In turn, a nurse would take her, then proceed with tube-feeding. While I had to trust that the nursing staff was acting in Jade's best interests, I couldn't help but feel like an incompetent mother or, more disheartening, just the person who gave birth to her.

By now, everything seemed so unnatural. My baby hadn't been brought to my room. I had to ask *permission* to pick her up. I was told *when* to return her to bed and, most unnatural of all, I couldn't even *feed* her.

Later, Martin came by to visit. While taking turns holding Jade in the nursery, we tried to determine what this horrible diagnosis might be. We gave up; it just wasn't fair to hold this precious being in our arms, trying to determine what was "wrong" with her. Martin concluded, "I'm sure there has been some terrible mistake; just wait and see." I could only hope that he was right.

We placed Jade back into her crib, kissed her a thousand times and, just as we were about to leave the nursery, Dr. O'Reilly called to find out how we were managing with all the worry. I began to panic and, at this point, pleaded for more information.

Dr. O'Reilly was as noncommittal as before. "The diagnosis," not yet specified, "could affect various organs of the body . . . the kidneys, liver, heart, brain . . ."

Trying not to cry, I asked, "When do you expect to give us the exact diagnosis?"

At that frightening point, probably more overwhelming than the actual diagnosis was the lack of facts on which to base all our worrying.

Dr. O'Reilly apologized and said, "Due to the long holiday weekend, certain tests have to be postponed for a couple more days. Once they're completed, we will require approximately one more week for the results to be confirmed."

It felt as though our lives were being put on hold due to a stupid holiday. The doctor then added, "I'd like to meet with you and your husband on Wednesday evening in order to give you more information. The information provided will answer most of your questions, it will be 99 percent accurate, and the confirmation will be available sometime next week."

Martin left me in my room of sadness and hopelessness. I started to cry again but really wanted to scream as loudly as I possibly could. I don't know why, but it was all I could think of. Perhaps screaming would rid my system of all this tension and worry, once and for all.

Though exhausted, I was reluctant to fall asleep because I might not wake up in time for Jade's next feeding, and I couldn't bear the thought of her gagging.

If ever I was going to be an optimist, today, July 3, was the day. I tried to steer my thoughts in the most positive direction possible. I suddenly had a very strong faith in medicine—I had to.

The thoughts that ran through my mind were horrifying, but whatever Jade's health problem, I was determined that there'd be a solution. In trying to imagine the worst possible scenario, but on a positive note, I concluded that if my baby's heart had some kind of defect, then the doctors could perform surgery and repair it. If her liver or kidneys were not functioning as they should, then the doctors could correct that as well. But if Jade's brain was damaged, God forbid, I knew that nothing could change that.

I had to stop contemplating the possibilities, as my optimistic thinking was taking a rapid turn for the worse.

Back in the nursery, Jade had the hiccups again. It didn't take much to keep me entertained: just seeing any movement at all in her little body was encouraging.

I picked her up and brought her into the adjoining visitors' room. Much to my relief and satisfaction, she responded well to my nursing her. Holding Jade in my arms was like a consolation in itself. I just prayed for some good news, prayed that everything would be fine, and that Jade would receive a clean bill of health. And if that were not possible, I prayed that whatever illness she might have, she would be cured.

Jade and I were then joined by a young nurse who pulled up a chair alongside us. In her arms she had a little baby whom she was preparing to feed. We talked a while, until I found the conversation was leading to a much-too-sensitive topic. This nurse asked me about my greatest fear, should there in fact be something wrong with my baby.

Horrified, I replied, "Brain damage."

She started telling me of her own personal experiences with mentally retarded children, but it was a topic that I just couldn't handle, at least not now. While the nurse emphasized how loving and affectionate these children really are, I sensed she knew something that I didn't. I started to cry as I blurted out, "Does my child have brain damage? Is that what you're trying to tell me?"

The nurse instantly became worried that she might have unintentionally revealed unauthorized medical information. She tried to assure me that she in no way intended to upset me, but rather, she wanted to impress upon me that should my greatest fear become a reality, it really wouldn't be such a horrible thing.

That afternoon, my mother, my sister Lynn, and my friend Wendy, came to visit. While observing Jade through the nursery's display window, I was trying very hard to hold back the tears, not wanting anyone to suspect that anything was wrong.

"She's cute!" "She's such a darling." "She's so tiny and beautiful." "What beautiful blue eyes!"

I delighted in the compliments, and that's all I wanted—compliments—no brain damage. I just wanted a normal, happy experience.

Back in my room, alone for the rest of the day, I tried to absorb all that was happening. I started to worry—not that I hadn't been all along—I just couldn't make any sense out of so much senselessness. My head was throbbing, I felt sick to my stomach, and I knew that aspirin wasn't going to cure any of these ailments. What I needed was good news.

CHAPTER TWO

On the day of verdict, I woke up feeling that my world was crumbling, as though God were somehow punishing me. I could hear other mothers from across the hall talking about the new addition to their families. I could hear how excited they were, as they laughed and exchanged their happy birthing experiences. I couldn't eat a thing. I just wished that everyone would shutup! I wanted someone to hurt just as much as I was; maybe then, I wouldn't feel so alone in this nightmare.

It was 11 A.M., and I hadn't yet gone to the nursery to see Jade. Somehow I thought it would hurt less if I didn't see her just then. That thought lasted but a few minutes when I knew that I just *had* to see her. Jade had already been fed and was now sleeping. I didn't wake her but placed my hand on hers and said a silent prayer.

I then decided to go to the regular nursery. I couldn't believe the size of the babies there! After spending all of my time in the Special Care Nursery, where there were mainly premature infants, these newborns looked like giant babies. Too heavy for me to hold anyway, I thought.

Who was I kidding?

Martin arrived at the hospital around 5 P.M. We were both extremely nervous entering the nursery. I awkwardly took Jade out of her incubator and brought her into the visitors' room, where the meeting with Dr. O'Reilly was to take place. With Jade in my arms, I was going to prove to the doctor that there was absolutely nothing wrong with my child.

When the doctor arrived, she suggested that I return Jade to her bed while we talked, but I refused. I wanted this doctor to see, touch, and maybe get a feeling for Jade—then let her dare give us any bad news. For some reason, I felt that Jade's presence might miraculously change the outcome of this meeting.

Martin had braced himself for the worst. I began to tremble and was on the verge of tears when the doctor began:

"I realize how worried you have been and I can understand it. However, before I go any further, I want you both to know that Jade's condition has nothing to do with you; neither of you could have prevented it, and neither of you are to blame. Although we are not 100 percent certain, after running some tests, we have determined that your daughter has Down syndrome."

"What's that mean?" I asked nervously.

"Down syndrome is a genetic disorder that usually occurs in about one in 1,500 births in women under thirty-five years of age, with the risk being higher for older women. This condition begins at conception, when the egg or the sperm introduces an extra chromosome into the zygote, so that each cell in the resulting fetus will also get one too many chromosomes. The extra genetic material slows cellular activity, thus causing mental and physical retardation."

The moment I heard the word "retardation," I started to cry and held Jade tighter until a nurse came along and carefully pried her from my arms.

Martin and I took the news so unbearably hard and, through it all, I had noticed that the doctor had wiped away a few tears of her own.

Dr. O'Reilly continued explaining her diagnosis, but only Martin was listening now. I grabbed a pillow and buried my head in it so I could cry as loud as I had to.

I managed to catch the last part of the conversation: "Jade will be much like any other child. She has the same basic needs, but she'll walk a little later; she'll talk a little later, and she'll go to a special school for handicapped children. But please be assured that you will not be alone. There will always be help along the way whenever you need it. There are services for the handicapped, special learning and stimulation programs, and a

11

whole array of other services."

In all, I don't know how much I absorbed, but I asked, "What about all those things you spoke about on the phone concerning the kidneys and heart and liver and . . . ?"

Dr. O'Reilly replied, "Oh, everything seems to be fine. Jade has been examined, and there seem to be no other apparent problems. Everything is functioning properly, and her heart sounds good."

"I guess that makes it good and bad news," Martin added.

Still trying to absorb this crushing, overwhelming news, I asked, "How could this have happened to me? I'm only twenty-two years old!"

"While studies show that women over thirty-five years of age tend to have a higher risk of having a child with Down syndrome, it can happen to any woman," the doctor answered. "Call it a fluke, or call it an accident of nature, it just happens."

The doctor then concluded, "I feel very confident in this diagnosis and, as I've explained before, there are still some further tests to run, but I'm 99 percent certain that Jade does in fact have Down syndrome. I will arrange for us to meet next week, and I will answer any other questions you may have."

"When can the baby come home?" I asked.

"Just as soon as she responds better to feeding and has gained some more weight," she replied.

I then requested that Dr. O'Reilly explain Jade's condition to whoever might be visiting us that evening.

Martin and I remained in the visitors' room long after the doctor had left. We had each other's shoulder to cry on and, for the first time in a long time, I felt really close to him. We had a common interest, a common concern—Jade was *our* baby.

Martin went to the cafeteria, and I headed back to my room. Waiting in the corridor were my mother, Lynn, and Wendy. I could see from the sad expressions on their faces that they had already received the news. All I could muster was, "But I love her so much." The four of us went to the nursery's display window to observe Jade, and the tension seemed to dissipate a little as we began to admire this adorable little infant, this sweet little creature whose body was twitching again from hiccups.

I recall telling my visitors that I was aware of two other Down syndrome babies in the nursery, and that I'd overheard the nurses mentioning one of the babies was not going home—ever. Apparently, the parents didn't want the child and decided to place him in foster care. Each of us was appalled that someone could stop loving their own child because he wasn't "perfect." I would later learn not to be so judgmental.

Martin came to join us, each of us totally enchanted and absorbed in Jade, her tiny limbs, her pretty ash blonde hair, and her beautiful, deep blue eyes. Jade, without even being aware of it, or maybe she was, had managed to touch everyone's heart.

I advised Martin that I couldn't face another night in the hospital. I was scared and needed to sleep in my own bed. I returned to the room to gather my belongings and began to weep as I held my baby's "going home" outfit.

It was like an autumn evening—cold, windy, and wet outside. As Martin and I walked toward the parking lot, I stared up at the hospital's seventh floor windows. In a moment of disbelief, I cried, "My baby's in there! I'm going home empty-handed! This is not supposed to happen."

When we arrived home, it felt as though we had just come home from a funeral. Martin headed to the upstairs flat of the duplex where his aunt and uncle and two cousins lived. He said he wanted to break the news to them.

I went into the little nursery, which I had so enjoyed decorating during pregnancy. I sifted through the dresser drawers, holding each article of clothing as a precious gift. The clothing even smelled like a baby. I looked over to the wooden cradle, which my father himself had built for his grandchild. Empty.

I was lying in bed trying to decide what today's date was. God, it is July 5! That means it is true. Everything that has happened is for real.

I turned to Martin, but he wasn't there. The alarm clock said eleven o'clock. I had overslept. Poor Jade—I had missed her morning feedings. I jumped out of bed and called out for Martin, then realized he had already left for work. I noticed that my nightgown was stiff from the breast milk that must have been leaking all night. I bathed, dressed quickly, and headed out the door.

The bus took forever to come. With two buses and the subway, it took a good hour and a half to get to the hospital.

Jade was in a sound sleep. How could anyone possibly sleep under fluorescent lighting with all the clattering and conversations going on? I wanted so badly just to wake her, bundle her up, and take her home.

A nurse reported that Jade had drunk a little milk today, though not enough to satisfy. Again, she had to be tube-fed.

When Jade awoke, I took over. I held her little body in my arms, changed her sleeper pyjamas, and then brought her into the adjoining room to nurse her. She wouldn't respond, concentrating instead on what was going on around her—a hopeful sign?

I overheard a couple of people talking in the background. "There are three mongoloids here. It's just incredible, all of them born within the same week, right here at the same hospital."

Mongoloids? That sounds horrible! Could they be referring to the three babies with Down syndrome? I'd heard the term "mongolism" before but never really knew what it meant.

When Jade fell asleep, I placed her back in her crib, then telephoned Dr. O'Reilly, whose office was at the Montreal Children's Hospital.

"Dr. O'Reilly, is my baby a mongoloid?"

"Yes," the doctor replied, "the term, 'mongolism,' is often used when referring to Down syndrome; however, it's really not a correct term to use. The word, 'mongolism,' is used because people with Down syndrome have similar facial features to Mongolian people—a flat face and slanted eyes."

She continued, "I personally dislike the term, and more and more professionals are discarding the label, as it is

14

stigmatizing and doesn't make any medical or ethical sense." She added, "And just think of how the people from Mongolia must feel! One insensitive person must have made up the word and, unfortunately, it stuck."

"How can people be so ignorant?" I asked. "Thanks for answering my question. I just had to know."

The doctor then asked, "How are you and Martin coming along?"

"Martin feels that he needs a lot of diversion, and he's decided not to miss any work."

"That's probably the best thing then. And how are you managing?"

"I'm worried sick about Jade. I have a headache that just won't go away. I can't eat and have trouble sleeping. What's worse is that Jade is hardly drinking anything. I hate using that mechanical breast pump but I'm so sore and haven't any choice. There are just so many emotions being stirred at the same time. Is this normal?"

"Under the circumstances," the doctor replied, "I'm sure it is, but if you wish, I can put you in touch with one of the hospital's social workers. You may find it helpful to talk to someone about your concerns."

I declined, at least for the time being. Then remembered: "Oh, by the way, Dr. O'Reilly, I saw some pamphlets with my name on it on the desk at the nursing station."

"Oh, come to think of it, that's right," she said. "The booklets are distributed to hospitals by a parents' support group. These parents have all gone through the same experiences as you and your husband. Hopefully, you will find the information helpful, and it may answer some of the questions that will probably arise concerning children with special needs."

Since Jade was still napping when I got off the phone, I strolled down the corridor to visit the giant babies. I still couldn't get over the size of them in comparison to the Special Care infants.

I returned to Jade. She was so alert, watching everything attentively. She clasped my finger and just stared at me. I changed her, then carried her to the next room, explaining, "Jade, the sooner you decide to eat, the sooner you get to go home. So *please* eat. I love you so much, and I need you home with me—now."

Jade drank a little of my milk, but not enough. She had to be tube-fed again.

Martin met me at the hospital, stayed a while, then we left at about eight o'clock that evening. "I still can't believe it," I said to him. "This all seems surreal, like maybe it's all a dream." All he could add was, "I wish it was."

When we arrived home Martin left me at the front door and headed upstairs to his uncle's place. "I'll be back later," he said. "I'd like to visit my aunt and uncle for a while."

"Fine," I said sarcastically, "I'm sure *they* could really use your support right now!"

I had been lying awake in bed for some three hours, waiting for Martin to return. I needed to talk to him—now. I started to worry again. Was this the way life was always going to be? Was this the way it's going to be when Jade is at home? Was this the kind of support I could expect?

The next morning I tried to force myself to eat breakfast, but couldn't. I then decided that I should at least drink something to help keep my milk production going—so I could nurse that stupid mechanical pump! I prepared a banana milkshake, sat down at the kitchen table, and began to read the booklets from the hospital. With words like "special needs," the material was quite comforting. After yesterday's rude awakening, I was almost expecting something like: "How to Train Your Mongoloid." Mongoloids. Freaks. It all sounded the same to me.

I took the bus at rush hour to hasten my travel time to the hospital. I wished that for once I could walk into the nursery and Jade would be awake. I handed the nurse a couple of baby bottles containing breast milk expressed the previous night and that morning.

"Has Jade taken any milk this morning?" I asked.

The nurse checked Jade's chart. "She took a bit from the bottle during the night, but then she had to be tube-fed, and tube-fed again this morning."

I waited for about an hour. Jade was still sleeping, but I decided to pick her up anyway. That's what I needed. I needed to hold this precious, warm, lovable baby in my arms to derive as much comfort as possible.

Martin met me later in the day. "Were you here all day?" he asked.

"Yes," I replied. "There's not much else to do. I just wish that Jade would stay awake for longer periods of time. Most of the day, I am just waiting for her to wake up and then, before I know it, she's asleep again. But it's worth the wait because I do get to hold her between naps."

I spent every day of the next two weeks at the hospital. I would cuddle Jade as often as possible, then Martin would usually join us by early evening. During those two weeks, Martin and I had a couple of appointments with the genetic specialist. Jade's blood tests showed that "translocation" was the specific cause of her extra chromosome. As the doctor explained: "Karyotyping was done on Jade, which revealed forty-six chromosomes with the presence of a 21-21 translocation, thus in fact, making her trisomic for chromosome 21."

"Could you please explain it in simpler terms?" I asked.

"In simpler terms, it means, in most cases, people with Down syndrome are found to have an extra chromosome, which results in forty-seven chromosomes, rather than the normal forty-six. This is called 'Trisomy 21.'

"After taking blood samples from Jade, a karyotyping—a thorough study of the chromosomes—was carried out. As you know, during fertilization, the offspring receives twenty-three chromosomes from the mother and twenty-three from the father. In studying Jade's karyotyping, it would appear that she does have the normal count of forty-six chromosomes. But in pairing up the identical sets of chromosomes, we found one that could not be matched. What happened is, during fertilization, an extra chromosome had latched itself onto another thus resulting in an actual count of forty-seven. Translocation is a rare occurrence and simply means the translocating of one chromosome onto another."

The specialist went on, "Because there is a possibility that either one of you might be the carrier of a translocator gene, I would urge you both to have karyotypes done. All it will require from you is a simple blood test."

Martin and I agreed to this advice, thanked the doctor, then left.

Our second visit to the genetic specialist was to obtain the results of our blood tests. We were told: "Karyotypes done on both of you are completely normal. Thus, the unbalanced translocation in Jade occurred *de novo* during fertilization." She added, "The risks of your having a second baby with Down syndrome, Gail, is higher than other women of your age, but still only in the order of one percent. Prenatal diagnosis via amniocentesis done at sixteen weeks gestation is available, with the option then of aborting an affected fetus."

With a look of disappointment on his face, Martin responded, "Oh, well, we just won't have any more kids, that's all."

I resigned myself. Why did I think someone was out to get me? Who the hell cares anyway?

No, I do care.

Jade was now twenty days old and still being looked after by hospital staff. When was life going to be normal? When was Jade going to be cared for by me, her mother?

The days at the hospital were painfully long. I seldom spoke to anyone. One afternoon, I went downtown for a change of scenery and also to kill some time until the next feeding. I passed by a pet shop and decided to go inside. There was a fairly large crowd of customers, and I was tempted to strike up a conversation with someone, anyone. I just wanted to talk about normal things, such as the weather, the cute animals, anything other than what I was feeling. I felt alone—all these people, and yet I felt alone.

I next stopped at a restaurant and ordered a vegetable

salad. One positive step, I thought. I could barely eat half of it, though. What a waste of good food and money.

I wandered through the streets of the busy downtown core. Everywhere I went, there were babies, babies, and more babies. One baby cried, and my breast milk instantly squirted out, right through my nursing pads, right through my nursing bra, and right through my blouse. I so desperately wanted to ask a mother if I could borrow her baby. God, did I feel stupid—and scared. Scared that I would start crying right there in the middle of the street for all the world to watch—this pathetic mother who couldn't even feed her own baby.

I walked back to the hospital, only to find that I couldn't bring myself to go inside. Not knowing what to do, I stood there in the entranceway. I just needed and wanted to cry. Wearily, I left for home, which seemed an endless journey. Every time I pictured Jade, and every time I thought of the diagnosis, I couldn't control the tears and had to get off the bus in order to avoid embarrassing myself. I ended up taking five buses rather than the usual two.

I went straight to bed, buried my head in a pillow, and screamed. For some crazy reason, the clock radio went off. I yanked out its plug and smashed the damned thing against the wall. Looking for something else to destroy, I realized that it was me who was being destroyed. I felt like a madwoman needing restraints. I needed to be restrained from myself and my thoughts and my worries and my sadness. I threw myself on the bed and cried until I was too exhausted to cry any more, then fell asleep.

When I woke up, the misery engulfed me. All these bad things couldn't possibly be happening. Jade was fine, wasn't she? We were going to be a happy family, weren't we? Why couldn't I honestly answer *yes* to all of this?

I started to reflect on life as it had been before Jade came along. I thought about how unhappy I was then, and I started to think about how unhappy I was now. I reflected on the feelings I had on the day I learned that I was pregnant. The news had left me feeling absolutely overwhelmed with mixed emotion. I was blissful because all along something, or someone, special was missing from my life, and I realized that that someone was here now. But the news also brought about sad, insecure feelings, because I already had serious doubts that my marriage would last very long at the rate it was going. What a naïve nineteen-year-old I was to have made the mistake of associating the word "marriage" with "happily every after."

What my husband and I had in common as teenagers no longer existed. We no longer shared any of the same interests. I had hoped that we would both change, or grow up, or develop interests that were at least marginally similar, but we didn't. He frowned upon any new interests I expressed and discouraged any new goals; even new friends were unwelcome at our home. It was as though Martin had already reached his life's goal: a wife with a paycheque; a house (albeit rented) with lots of new furniture; a top-of-the-line sound system, among other pricey toys; an expensive car, and jobs to keep us both paying for it. I never thought of materialism as a true goal, but simply a way to keep peace. I believed that once Martin acquired whatever he wanted, we would move on and set more meaningful goals. I had never imagined that this would be it—that life would stagnate—and if I tried to venture out of this comfort zone, it would create a lot of hostility, to the point that Martin resorted to verbal, and sometimes physical, abuse.

Looking back, the thought of divorce was an exit I entertained only briefly. I had a Catholic upbringing and was taught that marriage was for better or for worse, no matter what. I had no idea that things would only get worse. The mere mention of leaving my husband resulted in physical threats, and I could never be sure he wouldn't follow through on them. Even against all these odds, I had somehow hoped that our marital problems would be resolved *before* the baby's birth. This was not to be.

And now, in determining which direction Jade's life was to follow, I was forced to evaluate my own life in the here and now. It was a frightening feeling to know that Jade was going to be a part of Martin's and my unhealthy scenario. My worries no longer focused on my abilities as a mother having to cope with a handicapped child, but on my abilities as a likely *single* mother having to cope with a handicapped child. Would I be a mother who could be self-sufficient, responsible, and knowledgeable? A mother who could provide a good, healthy, stable environment?

I decided to set up an appointment with the social worker, through the referral that had been provided to me earlier on.

In the meantime, my sister Lynn had come over to visit and cooked a wonderful, nourishing vegetarian meal. It was comforting when family and friends showed their concern and thoughtfulness. A couple of my friends, Wendy and Johanna, sometimes dropped over to visit, and we'd try to talk about something cheerful, something other than what was happening. But we'd always end up in tears. Jade couldn't possibly leave our thoughts.

Martin accompanied me to see the hospital's social worker. I tried to confide in this total stranger, tried to explain the unexplainable. My insecurities. My fears. My greatest worry that maybe I wouldn't know how to take care of my baby. "I'm scared," I told her. "Jade is expected to be discharged from the hospital soon, and I just don't feel that I'm prepared."

"Prepared for what?" the social worker asked.

"I feel that there are certain problems at home that need to be resolved." I wanted to tell this person about everything I was worried about but felt ashamed and couldn't bring myself to confide in her.

The social worker broached the subject of foster care. She said, "If you feel that you both need some time for adjustments, then foster care could be an option."

"Could you please explain more?" I asked.

"What I mean is, Jade could be placed with a foster family who is willing and able to care for her for as long as required. This will allow you the time to make some necessary adjustments. I will put you in touch with someone at the Social Service Centre who could explain everything to you. If you wish, I'll arrange an appointment for this afternoon."

Martin and I later went to visit Jade. We each took turns holding her. At this point I was no longer trying to breast-feed. I had decided a few days earlier that it was just too painful—so much milk but no consistent relief.

After a couple of hours had passed, a nurse came into the visitors' room and politely suggested that we return Jade to her bed in order to maintain the schedule. In a soft voice, she said, "This little one of yours is feeding much better now, and it won't be long before you can take her home."

As I held Jade, she clasped my finger and stared into my eyes, as she had done so many times before. It was different this time, though. She squeezed my finger tighter, and I felt, or maybe imagined, she was trying to tell me something. Take me home, maybe? Oh, God, that very instinct was there! As I placed her back in her crib it just tore me apart to see those beautiful eyes, still staring at me.

As we were leaving the nursery, I panicked, "Oh God, Martin, what do we do?"

"We might as well keep the appointment with the Social Service Centre, and we'll decide then," he answered.

It was a cold, impersonal feeling to walk into an office building to discuss such a personal matter, a matter that could alter our lives forever. The intake social worker, Mrs. Williams, seemed like an intelligent, understanding person who, she assured me, was very experienced with situations such as ours. Somehow I managed to force myself to speak out, letting some of my concerns be known. Mrs. Williams nodded sympathetically, as though she understood exactly where I was coming from. How, I wondered, could she know this in such a short time? No matter, I eventually found myself quite at ease, as I told her what had been going on in our lives.

"Under the circumstances, your feelings are probably very normal," Mrs. Williams said. "You're both so young. I was told by the hospital that you may be considering temporary foster care for your child."

I hesitated. "I'm not sure what to do. What kind of home would it be?"

"Foster homes are well-screened as far as the environment and the family's capabilities are concerned. We try to find a

22

suitable home that will meet the needs of the particular child. In this case, it would have to be one very special family, a family who can share their time and love with a special child."

I looked at Martin and started to cry.

Mrs. Williams looked at me, and said, "Do this only if you feel that you both need the extra time to adjust." She then looked at Martin. "You have been very quiet during this meeting. How do you feel about your baby being placed in foster care?"

"Martin, please say something," I urged. "Say what you feel. Jade is not just my baby—she's ours!"

Martin replied, "It's Gail's decision. She can't go back to work, not with a baby who is sick." Sick? I took offence but kept my mouth shut, instead giving a disapproving glare. Why Martin seemed somewhat unresponsive to this situation, I didn't know. Since his feelings were never fully communicated to me, I could only speculate that he either worried about the possible restricted income, or he genuinely felt that I, as the mother and primary caregiver, was perhaps the one in the best position to make this decision.

Mrs. Williams was now looking back and forth from me to Martin, trying to clue in to anything she might have missed. She said, "So far, your only contact with Jade has been in a hospital setting, but I think that once you begin having contact with her in a natural setting, you will feel better about things. Should you decide to place Jade in foster care, just think of it as a time to readjust, while resting assured that Jade is in caring hands. We would seek a kind, loving family for Jade and, whenever you feel you are ready, you can bring her home."

We had the most important decision of our lives to make. Or, at least *I* had.

CHAPTER THREE

It got to the point where I had to avoid eye contact with one certain bedroom door—Jade's. Life became a never-ending nightmare.

Why? One simple question, but no simple answer. I was waking up in the middle of every night, wondering when God was going to give me the answer. Each prayer became an emotionally draining experience. One very real and frightening concern was: Did God do this to punish me? But I couldn't think of anything I might have done that was terrible enough to warrant this. Maybe He was punishing Jade—I couldn't stop searching my aching soul.

"God," I prayed, "maybe You don't love *me* but please, please love my baby. Don't punish her because of something I might have done. Please, God, answer me. Why did You do this to my baby? I love her so much."

My mind flashed back to the hospital scene where everybody was taking care of my baby, everybody but me.

Tired of all my restless tossing in bed, I got up, stumbled into the kitchen, and poured myself a glass of milk. I sat down at the table and began to read some more information from the booklets regarding children with special needs. My eyes were burning. I cried out of desperation, for I had questions but couldn't find any answers.

I tried to envision our future. I tried to honestly imagine myself raising and, most importantly, teaching this child. Am I qualified? I began to seriously question my capabilities as a mother—my ability to do what other mothers do, and more. I thought about the potential happy, fulfilling times but I also started to think more about our home environment. I hated this thought, so I thought about pretending instead. I thought about how easy it would be to pretend this was a perfect, or at least near perfect, family.

Maybe if I pretended long enough, things might really change. Maybe Jade would turn this unhappy marriage into a happy one, just by being here. Maybe. Maybe everything would just fall into place when we're together as a family. Maybe.

Or maybe not.

By August 1, Jade was placed in foster care. Mrs. Williams had telephoned to say that Jade was now ready to leave the hospital and that they had found a wonderful family who was more than willing to care for her. She advised, "The foster parents, Jim and Joan Pearson, have another foster child, a five-year-old boy with Down syndrome. They also have five children of their own, including two teenage daughters, two teenage sons, and a ten-year-old son." She went on, "Over the years, Jim and Joan have been of great assistance to our centre and, personally, I am extremely happy that it was this particular family who responded to our request for a home."

I had mixed feelings about the news. I was happy, of course, about the foster family, but I also felt very sad that a foster home had to be an option at all. I was becoming so impatient that life hadn't yet become normal.

"I guess I won't see Jade today, then?"

"You can if you want, Gail. If you wish, you can come with me to the hospital today, and together we can bring Jade to her new home. This will give you the opportunity to meet the foster mother."

I thought about it a while. "No, Mrs. Williams, I don't think I can do it. I know how much it's going to hurt. I always expected that *I* would be bringing Jade home—to my own home, not someone else's. Tell me more about the foster mother."

We spoke for another few minutes. Everything I had been told about the family was positive, and now I just had to find a way to accept all that was taking place.

During the course of the next week, I decided not to visit

25

Jade. I decided to use this time to meet with two other parents of a mentally handicapped child and to learn all I could, as soon as I could. I asked Martin to accompany me.

We met Kristen, a friendly, affectionate, four-year-old girl with Down syndrome. Now I was better able to understand what was meant by the "sweet disposition" of children with Down's. Unlike a couple of comments I had recently heard from kindly neighbours, children with Down syndrome do not have strange, moonlike homely looks. Kristen's facial features, rather, looked different. But she was still very pretty, with deep brown eyes and blonde hair held up in two little pigtails. She was dressed in a cute little pink jumpsuit, and her smile was vivacious as she excitedly gave us a tour of her bedroom.

Kristen's parents, John and Barbara, were informative, providing many instances and details: "Kristen learned to walk when she was two years of age. When she turned three years old, she was completely toilet-trained. Her speech, as you probably notice, is quite clear, and she is now learning to read simple words."

"What about your job?" I asked Barbara. "Did you have a career that you had to give up?"

"No," she replied, "I was completely prepared to stay home full-time with any child I'd have, but having a child with Down syndrome means getting involved, really involved. I became aware of how important a teacher I was when I became involved with the Infant Stimulation Programs, for example."

Barbara then went on to explain how these programs, usually run in a school setting, offered activities to stimulate cognitive, fine, and gross motor skills. "As with any child," she continued, "there are times that require extra patience, but my husband gives me terrific support. He pitches right in. He enjoys spending a lot of time with Kristen, and we both play equally important roles in her life. We share all of the responsibilities."

I suddenly had a twinge of envy as I listened to Barbara speak of their family life. I couldn't take my eyes off of Kristen. She was such a delightful child, dancing around, offering us a "cup-a-tea," and showing us her storybooks and new Frisbee.

26

It was one visit I was glad we'd made. While we were driving home, I couldn't stop talking about it. "Didn't they look happy, Martin? That little girl sure had a lot of energy, and she seemed pretty smart, too."

Martin remained fairly quiet, then said, "She was cute, Gail, but do you really want to stop working? Barbara says that her daughter requires a lot of time and work—like those training programs."

"To be honest, Martin, I don't know what to do any more. Obviously, I can't get a regular baby-sitter. I'd need someone who would really want to get involved. I'd probably end up having to stay home, but I'm also not sure whether we can manage financially with just you working.

What I deliberately avoided saying was, "I'm also not sure whether *I* can manage financially, should that be the case," but I wanted to avoid an argument.

My mind kept going back to Kristen. Then the parents. Then the family. The happy family. "Did you notice how happy they were?" I asked.

No reply.

We sat quietly for a few minutes, both of us trying to absorb whatever new information we were given.

"Martin, after that visit we just had, I think I'm less fearful now about Down syndrome. I think it's really starting to sink in that our child is just like any other child, except that she has special needs. She'll need more time in learning to walk and to talk. She'll need more time for many things, but Jade will learn—I know she will."

"Did you notice how happy they were?" I asked again.

After receiving no response, I added, "There's something really special about that family. I can't explain it exactly, but I just had a really good feeling while I was there. It was like, like everything was so natural; nothing was forced. They weren't *trying* to be nice to each other—they *were* nice to each other. That little girl seemed to be incredibly happy. They just seemed to be content with their lives, and it seemed to come naturally, like there was natural harmony in their lives. Oh, I don't know if I can explain it any better, but it was definitely different, a different kind of family.

Maybe we could be a family like them?" I asked hesitantly. No feedback.

I sat quietly the rest of the way home. Why I expected a miraculous and life-changing revelation, I don't know.

We went to visit Jade at her foster home. It was a large, beautiful home in an attractive suburb in the West Island. The foster mother, Joan, greeted us with a big smile. She showed us into the living room, then went upstairs to get Jade. As Joan was coming down the stairs with Jade, who was still fast asleep, she laughingly remarked: "Don't let her sleepiness fool you; Jade's sure got a good set of lungs. She really lets us know when she's hungry."

Mrs. Williams was right. It was a totally different feeling to visit Jade here, as opposed to the hospital. Jim and Joan, it was clear to see, were two very kind, loving people. It was a busy household, kids coming in and out, and all the while, Jade remained fast asleep. We would hold her, swing her a bit, play with her arms and legs and, still, she remained asleep. Finally, her eyes opened, and she just stared up at us. What a beauty!

As we were leaving, I handed Jade back to the foster mother. Surprisingly, I felt no pangs of jealousy, as I might have expected in seeing someone else care for *my* baby.

During our drive home, I explained to Martin that the next few days would be very important—a critical time for us to reflect on all that we'd learned, and to have some serious discussions about our relationship and how we could make things better for all of us. But we quickly learned that we did not have the same priorities. One important thing, which we mutually reconfirmed, was that we both loved Jade. The other important thing we had reconfirmed was that *I* felt our relationship needed a guaranteed improvement in order to provide the kind of home that Jade, or any child for that matter, would need. I persistently stipulated the need for such a guarantee but, like so many times before, we ended up in a heated argument.

The following week we had an appointment at the Social Service Centre. A social worker, Carolyn, was assigned to follow up our case. "How are things going with you both?" she asked. "Have you been able to make some adjustments?"

First I turned to Martin, then to Carolyn, and said, "No, we have not. Martin and I just don't see things the same way, and we can't agree on what would make a good home for Jade." I didn't care that I was airing our dirty laundry; I simply didn't care about any of that anymore. There were just too many important issues at stake.

Carolyn looked at us, analytically, I think. "Obviously you both need more time to work things out. Why don't we meet again in another week."

We went to visit Jade. It was always a warm, comforting feeling just to hold her. Strange how Martin and I could agree on at least one thing. With so many unresolved problems at home, we had at least one thing in common—one little person whom we both loved.

In my eyes, Jade was now becoming more and more a part of her foster family. At least here, I thought, there is stability. I didn't hear constant put-downs. Nobody was being shoved up against the wall with a threatening fist at their face, no doors were slamming, nobody was shouting, no cars were screeching down the road. In fact, there was nothing here that even closely resembled any of the unspeakable things that went on in our house.

I never left Jade without first telling her that I loved her, and I truly hoped that she knew it.

A few days later, I went on my own to see Carolyn. I informed her that after careful deliberation, I was thinking about long-term foster care, or possibly even adoption. I started to sob.

"I want my baby to have no part of this mixed-up, unhappy place. I want to give her the best, even if I can't give it to her myself."

"It's so obvious how much you love your baby," she said, "but somehow I don't think that you really want to do this."

"Of course I don't *want* to do this. You don't understand—I *have* to do this. You just don't understand, and I can't explain it; there's just no point."

"What about Martin?" she asked. "Is this a mutual decision?"

"Yes, in a way it is. You see, Martin has already made his decision; that is, he chose to abide by mine. After lengthy, going-nowhere discussions about how I would like to improve our home life, we finally agreed on one thing: that it would be in Jade's best interests to place her in a good, secure, loving home—but the final decision would be mine."

"Well then, Gail, both you and Martin will have to return in order to sign consent forms. If you are serious about giving your child up for adoption, then you should be preparing yourself to let go, which means having no more contact with Jade." Those words were unbelievably crushing.

I started to cry. "I can't do that just now. I need to see her. And I just said I was *thinking* about adoption. But I will prepare myself either way. I'll just have to keep reminding myself of the benefits Jade will receive if she is being raised in a healthier, happier environment."

I occasionally went to visit Jade, sometimes with Martin, and often without. The foster family had since moved to town, so travelling was more convenient. I was never quite sure what Jade's foster family might have thought or exactly what information they had received from the Social Service Centre; all I knew at that point was that each visit was creating a lot of heartache.

Martin and I had decided to postpone our consent to any possible adoption for the time being, just in case our situation should change, but I personally was not optimistic.

I received a letter from the genetic specialist, which read:

> I am writing to you to correct part of the information which I gave you in our last meeting. Since your baby, Jade, has Down syndrome by virtue of having an unbalanced 21-21 translocation, which is due to a chromosomal rearrangement, as opposed to a true

Trisomy 21 with forty-seven chromosomes, you are, therefore, *not* at a higher risk of having a second child with Down syndrome. In view of this, prenatal diagnosis is not necessary but is available if you have sufficient concern.

I regret the error I accidentally made in our counselling session and hope that it has not needlessly upset you. Please do not hesitate to call if you have any questions.

After reading this, I thought, believe me, having another baby was the furthest thing from my mind.

Martin's reaction to this letter was, "This means we *can* have another baby!"

"No, Martin," I said, "this means nothing at all, not a thing. Don't even think it. We have a baby and, in case you've forgotten, she is living in foster care, because *we* are not suitable parents." His eyes were open, but I couldn't make him see.

My relationship with Martin wasn't improving in any way. We communicated less and less as time went on, except for criticisms. "Gail, you're not just going to mope around the house from now on, are you? Go back to work. We need the money, and I don't intend to support you while you're fully capable of working. Do something! Use your brains and find something."

"Martin," I cried, "How can I go back to my job and deal with everyone and their inevitable questions? I just can't handle it."

"Then find somewhere else to work," Martin demanded.

"All right, all right, I promise I'll get a job soon."

By a stroke of luck, within days, I found employment at a large pharmaceutical company. I worked in a laboratory, analyzing ampoules of medication, which was very clean and quiet work, requiring a lot of concentration. After I was trained, I worked alone and later realized that it was probably the worst thing for me. It was just too quiet, and my thoughts would constantly drift back to Jade. It often got to the point where I couldn't accurately analyze the ampoules due to the tears impairing my vision—fortunately, my work had to pass a final inspection. It required tremendous effort to concentrate on anything but thoughts of Jade.

Martin was quite content now, as I was out working every day and bringing home a much larger paycheque than I had in my previous job. I felt like a zombie. Was this it? Have a baby, give her up, and then continue on with life, as though the baby never existed?

After pleading with Martin to agree to my quitting my job, I finally did so. He didn't approve, but I no longer cared. I knew the loss of income would create a lot of loud arguments and punishment, but I just didn't care anymore. I hated this death sentence I was serving. I hated the long hours at work where I was thinking only of Jade. I hated the fact that I was too ashamed even to let my family and friends know about the situation. I truly hated everything about everything.

Over the next few months Martin was growing more bitter, and I knew that I was greatly to blame because, after all, I no longer cared about anything or anyone, except Jade. I felt like my life was veering out of control, and I was just letting it happen.

When Martin went out, sometimes he'd inform me where he was going, and when I could expect him to return. "I don't care," was my typical response. I knew I was turning into a cold-hearted bitch, but maybe, hopefully, he would leave me or, better still, maybe he'd allow me to leave him, with no financial burdens, or physical threats.

Martin and I met with the social worker and informed her of our decision. We did not officially consent to adoption, but we were open to learn of any possibilities of a good home, at least for us to consider. In the meantime, we consented to Jade's placement in long-term foster care. We told the social worker that our decision had been carefully deliberated and that we were prepared to abide by it. We were also preparing ourselves to let go completely, permitting Jade to be raised by her foster family, without any interference on our part.

We brought Christmas gifts to Jade when we went to say our final good-bye to her. What made things a little easier was the fact that she did not even know us, at least not as her parents. To Jade, we were just visitors.

It was an evening I'll never forget. Jade had just learned to roll over, and she was rolling around on the living room carpet. Emmanuel, the other foster child, was kissing Jade and playing with her. What had struck a heartwarming chord was seeing Emmanuel and Jade together, just like brother and sister. Jade's eyes lit up when Emmanuel was around. It brought back a feeling, but a feeling that belonged to someone else. I thought about John, Barbara, and Kristen.

I thought of the natural harmony for which I'd been yearning. But it was right here, right now, and Jade was an integral part of it.

I returned home to continue life in my "moping" mode, as Martin called it, and I can't say that he was wrong. I spent so much time alone. I missed Jade terribly and often wondered about her. She was no longer a part of my life, but a child of another family. God, it hurt so much!

The pressure was on again: "Gail, get a job or move out!"

Did I hear right? Move out? There were no threats this time. I would definitely take that into consideration, providing there were no strings attached. "If I go, Martin," I insisted, "I need to know that I won't have any bill collectors coming after me for the loans I co-signed. As soon as the last loan is paid off, I'm out of here. Guaranteed!"

All I could think about throughout each and every day was Jade, and my unhappiness. It was possibly becoming an obsession.

Martin and I were growing more distant, if that were possible, as time slowly drifted by. In a way, however, I had to admire him, because at least he was able to deal with his feelings and get on with his life, whereas I was stuck in a place somewhere between limbo and hell. We were no longer a couple, and hadn't been in a long time. We were in every true sense of the words, living separate lives.

I had no zest for life and was becoming more and more depressed. I came to the painful realization that things were not ever going to change for the better. I was never going to see Jade again and, therefore, I could not foresee any purpose in my life. I was dead, or maybe it was wishful thinking.

I could walk; I could talk when I had to; my heart was still beating. Sometimes I'd eat, an annoying but necessary task, as I impatiently forced myself to chew, then swallow, waiting for my growling stomach to shut the hell up. No matter what I ate, the taste, the smell, and the texture were all the same—bland. The only moments of contentedness were sleeping moments, since sleep offered opportunities of hope. I would take my fantasies to bed, hoping that if I thought about them long enough, they would come to be realized in my dreams.

And sometimes they were. Sometimes Jade and I would take a nice leisurely stroll through some lush green forest trails. Sometimes we'd play on a sandy beach on some tropical island. Sometimes we'd read books under the weeping willow tree right next to our log cabin, and sometimes we'd just snuggle in the grass under the warm sun.

But the moment I awoke, the hopes disappeared, and I had to face the world again. I'd be awakened with a chastising remark about how lazy I was. I'd lie and say that I only had a couple hours sleep the previous night, and that I had been literally running around doing errands all day. I'd wait until the coast was clear before returning, with my fantasies, to the single bed in the spare room. I never even took the time to consider what a terrible wife I was. I had no desire to speak with my husband; I had no desire to go out with him, not that I had been invited; I had no desire to prepare dinner for him, and least of all, I had no desire to sleep with him.

While Martin was out one evening, I decided that I wanted to go far away, so far that even I wouldn't know where I was. I hated this world and wanted to get away from it, if only for a while.

I had some tranquilizers that were prescribed months ago

34

for my insomnia, but which had never been used, since I'd rather lose sleep than worry about addiction. I don't know how many pills I swallowed, or how much vodka I drank, or how much hashish I smoked—the leftovers from Martin and his friends. All I knew was that the bad feelings were becoming less and less intense, to the point that I didn't want to feel anything anymore. I was very relaxed and no longer crying. I was no longer feeling. It was a relief.

I could hear a faint ringing, even though the phone was nearby. Maureen, a friend of mine, called to chat and tried to encourage me to resume my career in the field of machinery and equipment appraisals. She tried to convince me that my co-workers would understand, but I could only envision looks of pity. She then sensed that something was terribly wrong and contacted my parents.

At some point, Martin came home. I was stooped over the toilet bowl, trying to vomit, and crying, "I'm going to die, I'm going to die!"

Martin grabbed my arm and dragged me over to the living room couch. "What the hell did you do?" he yelled. "You are so incredibly stupid!"

From that moment on, I was merely an onlooker. Somehow I had completely detached myself from this situation. I was not a part of this experience. It was as though I had floated outside of my body. I floated up toward the ceiling and looked down at what was happening. Martin was still yelling at me—the physical me. With sheer hatred, I watched over him and decided that I wanted no more of this. I didn't want to come back to this hellhole!

(I later learned through a television documentary and written articles on the subject, that some people claimed to have had near-death experiences. It was something that really hit home with me, a real eye-opener. I would have never thought it possible. In view of my own experience, however, I guess I had to believe it, or at least part of it. But I never felt the warmth, or the glow, or the love, or the gleaming light at the end of the tunnel like the others did—because if I had felt any of those feelings, or had seen any of those things that even resembled love, I surely would have followed that path, running as fast as my legs could take me.)

Maureen, her husband, and my parents had arrived. Everybody was rushing to get me—the physical me—to the hospital. Maureen, I later learned, had made every effort to keep me alive. While I was unconscious, or near unconsciousness, she pinched and slapped me. At that point, she figured, the only thing I could respond to was pain, and she was right.

I cried, "Where's my baby?"

The doctors at the hospital succeeded in reviving me, and I felt so foolish and embarrassed by the whole scene.

At my parents' urging, Martin and I went to their house. Trying to be helpful to Martin and me, my father pointed out that I really needed to take better care of life.

"Think of what you've put Martin through."

And he was right. I apologized to Martin. I apologized to my parents. I apologized to Maureen, and I apologized to her husband. I was apologizing so much that I almost forgot how I ended up in this predicament in the first place.

With my parents' words of encouragement, I somehow managed to resolve some of my negative attitudes toward life. Privately, however, I held certain conditions for myself. I knew at this point that my marriage could not be saved, but I was determined to work out a better life for myself. I realized that without a goal, I could not survive.

I was determined now, more than ever, that someday, somehow, Jade and I would be together again. My fantasies *would* be realized. She and I *would* be our own family. That became my goal, and that became my reason for being.

CHAPTER FOUR

I promised myself that from now on life would only get better. It had to. I could no longer endure this feeling of being buried alive in a deep, dark pit. Instead, I resolved to haul myself out, a goal that at first seemed unachievable. But it turned out to be easier than I ever imagined possible.

By March 1980, I was employed in a secretarial position and, though I exaggerated my qualifications, I was confident that I could easily handle any job I chose to handle. I would learn accounting, production control, and office management. That was the new me!

I developed a much happier and healthier attitude toward life in general. Martin and I seldom argued any more, but then again, we seldom saw each other. It was no longer important to me that Martin and I were so different, because I knew that someday I was going to strike out on my own—just as soon as the last loan was paid off. The time factor didn't seem to matter either. All that mattered was that I was actually planning a future, and it was of utmost importance that everything be perfect for Jade. I had to be a realist. I had to be responsible and make certain that financial burdens were lifted, since I wanted nothing to stand in the way of our mother-daughter reunion. I didn't want anything hanging over me, except the sun and the stars—and God.

Any new acquaintance I made, either through my job or socially, never suspected that I even had a child, and I kept it that way. There was no point, I figured, in revealing my private life, and I decided to keep it secret until the day that things were to change.

It was wonderful. I suddenly had a zest for life, a true ambition: Jade and I were someday going to be together. That was my goal, my means of survival!

In June, I remembered—not that I could ever forget—Jade's first birthday was coming up, and I started to make plans. I got up early one Saturday morning and made a list of all the things I thought a one-year-old would like to have. I spent the day going from shop to shop. I was trying to imagine what Jade would look like in certain outfits that I picked out. How big was she, I wondered? Everything I bought had to be tastefully selected, for these gifts were for *my* little girl.

I hadn't wrapped the gifts right away, because I wanted to spend a little time each day examining the clothes and trying to imagine how Jade would look in them. I'm sure if I had told this to anybody, they probably would have thought my behaviour slightly odd, to say the least, but I cherished anything that was associated with Jade.

A friend of mine delivered the gifts to Jade on her birthday. Except for Jade's foster mother, whom I'd eventually confide in, nobody else knew of my future plans—not the social worker, not my parents, and not my friends. I figured I'd let them know when the time came, and I so looked forward to that time. Anyway, I think I must have cried the entire day on July 1, missing Jade so much and yearning to hold her.

Ever since the last day I visited Jade in foster care, I had continually been in touch with the social worker and occasionally I telephoned Jade's foster mother directly. It was those conversations that kept me going, a constant reinforcement. "Jade is doing great! Jade has learned a new word. Jade has started to crawl." And whenever I learned of her progress, I too progressed.

On November 12, my curiosity just had to be satisfied. Without informing Martin or the social worker, I went to visit

Jade. It was like a dream come true. She was exactly how I had imagined her. She had pretty blonde hair, and her eyes were as bright as ever. She had the most radiant smile—she was simply adorable!

Joan had mentioned that Jade was a bit stubborn. I giggled, knowing full well where she might have gotten that trait. "She has a mind of her own," Joan said. "One cannot force her to do anything she doesn't want to do." What an afternoon! I still couldn't believe that I was there—with Jade.

When I was on the bus returning home, I wanted to scream out and tell everybody who it was I had just seen. I'm sure I must have had a smile from ear to ear—I was so utterly happy!

Martin wasn't home yet, and I wasn't sure whether or not to tell him of my visit. I was only sure of one thing—that I didn't ever want to forget this afternoon.

The following day I received a telephone call from Carolyn, the social worker. "I heard you visited Jade yesterday," she said. "Why hadn't you informed me that you were going to visit? I think you should have had some counselling first."

"It took a long time for me to build up the courage to visit," I answered, "and the last thing I would have needed was for you to say exactly that—that I would need some counselling first."

"You should have advised me in any case, Gail. As you know, Jade's foster parents have made a long-term commitment, and I wouldn't want you to jeopardize anything."

"Jeopardize! How do you suppose I would jeopardize Jade's foster care?"

"I simply mean that everything is going very smoothly. The foster parents are happy, and Jade is happy, and I don't think you should interfere. Besides, you can't just start visiting Jade again without letting me know. I need to have a meeting with my superiors to see if they approve of this situation."

"Listen, Carolyn, I am Jade's mother. I am not interfering, but I happen to love Jade very much, and I do not need you to tell me what I can and cannot do. And I fully intend to visit Jade again at Christmastime, or sooner, with or without your approval. By the way, Carolyn, aren't you supposed to be helping me with changing my situation, so that maybe this whole arrangement with Jade could change? I have plans, you know." Then I kept quiet. I sure didn't want her to know about my plans for fear that she would discourage me.

Carolyn lightened up. She put on a sweet telephone voice and asked, "Gail, would you like me to go with you? I haven't seen Jade in such a long time, you know, and I would really like to see her."

"Bullshit!" I felt like saying. "No thank you, Carolyn. I would prefer to visit Jade by myself." I certainly didn't need anyone telling me how to act or how to feel or when to leave, or anything.

When I hung up the phone, I muttered, "What a bitch!"

"Who was that?" Martin asked as he walked into the kitchen. "Nobody," I replied. "Just a half-brained social worker who is insinuating that I might be jeopardizing Jade's foster care."

"What?" he asked.

I hesitated, then said, "Oh, never mind." After further thought, I said, "Martin, I want to see Jade at Christmastime. I want to bring her some Christmas presents. Do you have a problem with that?"

"No," he replied, "are you sure it's not going to be too difficult a visit?"

"No, I'm definitely sure."

I saw Jade a few days before Christmas. She was very shy toward me, and why shouldn't she be? To Jade, Joan was her mother—not me. Jade wouldn't even allow me to look at her, let alone try to hold her. When I made any attempts, she pulled away and screamed. One would think that I was trying to torture her. But whether she was screaming or not, I was determined to cuddle her before my visit was over.

It was so funny to see Jade crawling around on the carpet. She picked up a tiny thread, almost invisible to the naked eye, and handed it to Joan. When Joan left the room for a moment, Jade

40

quickly followed behind. One day, I thought, it will not be this way. One day Jade will be as happy and as comfortable with me as she is now with Joan. It was now getting dark so I thought it best to leave. Before leaving, I handed Joan the bag of gifts, along with a Christmas card, which read:

Dearest Jade,
Even though we are apart
I feel as though we're near
And I've a special little secret
To softly whisper in your ear:

On this coming Eve of Christmas
When the world is fast asleep,
Someone is going to come
And put presents under the tree.

They say his name is Santa,
The husband of Mrs. Claus,
And when he looks in on you
He will most certainly pause.

He'll see a pretty little baby,
Pretending to be asleep,
But, hush, do not tell him,
Try not to make a peep.

It might ruin his little surprise,
Should you let him know,
So best wait till he's gone,
Continuing his journey through the snow.

And on his continued journey,
He promised to stop by my place,
To leave an imaginary picture
Of the smile upon your face.

I'll look forward to falling asleep,
Just to hold you in my dreams,
And it'll only be "us"
Just you, my precious, and me.

And when we all wake up
Christmas will be here
And I wish you every happiness
Today and throughout the year.

Loving you, as always,
Gail

One evening in January, I telephoned Joan to see how Jade was doing and received some terrible news. "Gail, has anyone from Social Services been in touch with you?" Joan asked.

"No," I replied. Now I was beginning to worry.

Joan explained, "Jade was very sick during Christmas. She had what appeared to be a cold, but when we noticed that her lips, fingertips, and toenails were turning a bluish colour, we brought her to the hospital."

She went on, "A cardiologist named Dr. Gibbons examined Jade, and it was discovered that she has an enlarged heart. Apparently, this heart defect was existent at birth, but it went undetected. There is a hole in her heart that prevents the blood from circulating properly. Because of this defect, hypertension has developed in her lungs.

Unfortunately, nothing can be done. Surgery, I am told, would be too risky. The doctors cannot determine at this time exactly what the condition means in terms of physical activity, and Jade's heart problem will have to be closely monitored at regular intervals."

I just couldn't find any words. Joan continued, "I'm sorry to have to be the one to tell you this, and I'm surprised that no one from Social Services has informed you."

When I got off the phone, I was still trying to absorb all her words. Irreparable heart defect. My poor baby, I cried. My poor, poor, precious baby! I was grieving all over again, only this time it hurt so much more.

I made an appointment with Dr. Gibbons, who confirmed all that Joan had told me. I was scared to ask but had to anyway. "What about Jade's life expectancy?"

"There is no clear answer on that," the cardiologist replied. "Each case is entirely different, but with proper care and consistent monitoring, who can say? We'll just have to do our very best in caring for Jade and hope for a bright future."

That's all I can do, I decided.

That night I woke up in a cold sweat. I bolted upright and switched on the lamp. Almost dazed, I looked around the room, trying to determine whether I'd been dreaming. It was all too confusing. Since Jade's birth I'd had so many dreams, fantasies, and nightmares that often the real facts didn't register straight away. Then I remembered. It was real. I started to cry.

"Oh God! How could You do this? Haven't You done enough already? Jade is *my* baby. Do You enjoy seeing people suffer? How could You do this to my baby? Answer me!"

As usual, no reply.

In February, I told Martin that I was leaving him. Life was, or could be, too short. I explained, "The last of our debts will be paid off by the end of next month, and I'll be financially ready to live on my own." "Well, then, go!" he shouted. "As I've told you before, you'll never make it on your own, you'll see!"

I protested, "If I chose to continue living the way you do, of course I wouldn't make it. By living with you, I've learned how *not* to live! I'm through with paying your loans, and I will never, ever, owe money to anyone."

It was a month of hell. Martin was either pleading with me to stay with him, as he didn't want to lose my paycheque, or he was cursing at me to leave him now, at that very minute—even though I hadn't anywhere else to go.

One night, in a fit of rage, he threw all of my belongings out of the bedroom closet and dresser drawers. He took a sledgehammer and proceeded to smash a couple of bedroom lamps. He glared at me with such hatred that I knew I was next.

I stood in the corner of the bedroom, with nowhere to run. My legs shaking and heart pounding violently, I was sure he was going to kill me. I was sure that I was going to become just another statistic on a long list of fatal domestic disputes.

Then, for a fleeting moment, Martin looked just as terrified as I was. Tears began to roll down his face as he told me, "Just go! I'm sorry, Gail," he cried. "You'd better leave now, because I came *so* close to killing you. Life was just so much easier when you accepted everything the way it was. Go now, while you still have the chance."

He then dashed out the door and screeched off in his car. At that horrible moment in time, I don't know that I would have even cared if the car had crashed.

In a shaking panic, trying to determine where I should go, I called a taxi. At about 9 P.M. I arrived at the church's rectory where I was greeted by the parish priest who, incidentally, was the same priest who had married Martin and me just a few years earlier. After I described the night's events, the priest strongly urged me to leave Martin immediately, and he offered to help me to find a place to live. In the meantime, I stayed at a friend's place.

CHAPTER FIVE

From my parents' roof, to my husband's roof, and now, finally, I had my own roof. For a fresh start, I rented a charming, spacious, one-bedroom flat that had hardwood floors and some original woodwork intact. Consisting of only four units, the building was located in Crawford Park, a small residential part of town. From any window I chose to look out, I had a beautiful view of the St. Lawrence River, which would be lined with lush greenery and flowers when summer came.

With such a cozy place to live, I thought, who needs furniture? I did, however, collect a few basics: a simple bookcase and a corner hutch that my father had built, an oak kitchen table my brother David had built, and a futon I had purchased. I was thrilled when a friend gave me his old stereo and a small television. The kitchen sink was the old-fashioned deep tub kind, perfect for doing laundry. Large cushions completed the living room setting. I used a tree stump for a coffee table, and dishes, lamps, and so forth were easy enough to obtain at thrift shops.

I felt like a flower yearning to grow. I got a second emotional wind and started to feel very comfortable and good about myself. When I wasn't working or at evening accounting classes, I was outdoors taking long leisurely walks and enjoying a sense of freedom that I hadn't known in a long time, if ever. Other times, I was preoccupied with reading or, I should say, studying. I wanted to learn as much as I could about children with Down syndrome and to discover useful ways of helping them to learn. I felt emotionally stronger with each passing day; I enjoyed the tranquility and the fact that I no longer had anyone yelling at me, swearing at me, running my life, or criticizing my actions. I realized that I did have control of my life. Total control. And I could make *anything* happen. God, what had taken me so long to learn this?

Despite feeling more and more confident with each passing day, I still experienced episodes of insecurity and fear that my ex-husband, in a spate of jealousy, might come around and in some way try to ruin my newfound happiness.

My downstairs neighbour, Mr. Gibbons (no relation to the cardiologist), was a sweet, gentle man in his early eighties. His wife had passed away about a year before. When I first moved into the building, I mentioned to him that I was a little nervous about living alone. Over time, I introduced him to any friends who visited me, and he'd always let me know if someone stopped by while I was out.

I don't know why, but as long as I could see people going about their lives in the brightness of day, I could never imagine anything bad happening. My greatest worries—fears that something horrible might happen—would overtake me in the darkness of night, and I'd lie awake while the rest of the world was asleep.

I pictured worst-case scenarios, then tried to make a plan of action. At night, I'd remember Martin's threats. What if he had a really bad day and broke into my house to make good on them? Or what if one of his shifty friends showed up to do the job for him? What if I couldn't get to the phone in time?

Sometimes I'd hear a car engine idling in the street. With my heart pounding, I'd quickly double- and triple-check the locks on the doors and windows. Nights like those seemed endless, but at last the alarm clock would sound, and I'd welcome the light of day.

Ultimately, without too much detail so as not to overly concern him, I told Mr. Gibbons that I didn't feel safe at night. We then came up with a perfect plan of action: three sharp knocks on my floor meant, "Call the police."

Just knowing that someone was looking out for me helped to dispel my nighttime fears, and I finally began to feel secure.

At night I often thought about Jade—what would it be like to see and hold my precious little baby again? I held my values so dearly and realized that I now had the environment I'd been striving for. It was an environment that I'd be proud to share with my child. I was also proud of the fact that since leaving Martin, I had come a very long way in a relatively short time.

I was so grateful for my good fortune that I wanted to thank the whole world; then I realized who was probably responsible. I figured that if I could yell at Him, accusing Him of abandonment and callousness, then it was only fair that His generosity now be acknowledged.

I started to visit Jade on a regular basis. She was now an adorable little toddler, often dressed in pretty little outfits, her long hair done up in two pigtails. She wore corrective eyeglasses to help strengthen her eye muscles, and actually, she looked pretty cute, like a real intellectual.

Although I thoroughly enjoyed my weekly visits with Jade, they weren't without disappointments. Joan had once told me that Jade wanted nothing to do with anyone she hadn't known for at least a year. Apparently, that's how she reacted to both of Joan's daughters' boyfriends. But I accepted Jade's terms, for I expected that with time and patience, she would learn to accept me.

It was a whole new exciting life. The immediate goal was for Jade and me to get to know each other better, then to spend our weekends together. And Jade, I thought, if you don't agree, that's just too bad. I've waited too long for this.

Jade's second birthday was coming up, and it was the first time that I could actually choose some outfits and know exactly what size to get.

Joan's whole family had been very understanding and supportive. Jade simply adored her foster father. She also adored her foster brothers, Myles, Lorne, and Danny, and it was obvious how Margaret and Anmarie loved Jade. And, of course, there was

Emmanuel, whom Jade liked to boss around. They were great pals.

While organizing my life into this satisfying order, I realized that I still had a few loose ends to tie. My marriage, I was well aware, had to be legally terminated. After speaking with my parish priest, I had learned that an annulment would not be possible without the involvement of family and friends; hence, I chose to find a lawyer instead.

On grounds of spousal abuse, the divorce proceedings were started, and Martin was served with the petition. During a subsequent telephone conversation with him, I was told that he wasn't going to contest the divorce, providing I didn't ask for financial support, or anything else. *A small price to pay for freedom.* From then on, all ties were severed. Other than the odd bit of news, such as Martin's involvement in a new relationship, and his move to another house, I hadn't heard, nor was I interested in, any updates.

Working all week had greater rewards than just a paycheque, for I knew that come Saturday, I would be seeing Jade. She had such a funny character, and she so enjoyed making people laugh.

She didn't walk yet. She literally "bummed" around. It was so amusing to see this little kid getting around on her bottom, and she was so fast. The knees of her pants never wore out, just the bum part. It was a convenient way for her to get around, since crawling meant having to use her arms whereas bumming around offered the convenience of carrying toys and things wherever she wanted to go. Smart kid!

She had a very small vocabulary, but some words were amazingly clear. In every way Jade was just so delightful. Anmarie once told me about how Jade liked to start every morning with kisses. On awakening, she'd poke her head toward the bar of her crib and pucker up, waiting for a kiss. Then she'd go to each and every rung, expecting another kiss.

Jade was comfortable with me around, providing that Joan was also present, but the minute Joan disappeared into another room to allow Jade and me some privacy, Jade would protest. She

48

would cry frantically and, I have to admit, sometimes it really hurt. On the bus journey home, it was all I could do to keep from bursting into tears.

Eventually, Joan and I decided that the best way to solve this problem was to give Jade no alternative. I'd come to the house, put Jade in her stroller, and off we'd go to the park. Whenever I talked to Jade, she'd peek at me out of the corner of her eye, giving me the dirtiest look. She certainly had an effective way of letting me know that my presence was not appreciated. And if she didn't want to see me at all, she'd simply close her eyes for the longest time, perhaps hoping that I'd disappear.

As Joan and I had discussed, as soon as Jade was more comfortable with me, it would then be a good time to start taking her home for weekends. But Jade truly had a mind of her own. I'm sure she must have thought, *I'm not going to make things easy for Gail. It's more challenging this way.*

It was October 1981, and this Thanksgiving weekend truly was a time to give thanks. I explained to my friend, Steve, that I needed his moral support this coming Saturday, the first day I was going to take Jade home with me. Steve gladly obliged, drove me in his car to pick up Jade, and agreed to spend the day with us. While I was emotionally preparing myself to handle Jade's inevitable screams and tears, I was pleasantly surprised to find none. Jade trusted me, she actually trusted me! With this grateful thought in mind, I thanked Steve and told him that his support probably wouldn't be necessary after all.

Steve left Jade and me at my front door. "Call me when Jade needs to be driven back," he said.

As I carried Jade up the stairs to my place, I thought she'd scream and cry as soon as we got into the house. But she didn't and, instead, bummed her way into the living room to make new discoveries, such as records, books, cassettes, stationery, and my typewriter. She then bummed her way into the kitchen where she found cupboards, pots, pans, plastic bowls, and so on.

"Jade," I said, "you mean this is all there was to it? You mean I'd been visiting you all this time, just waiting for you to feel more secure with me, and this is all it took? You mean, all I had to do was kidnap you in order for you to be comfortable with me?"

While pointing to an upper cupboard, Jade responded, "Wassat?"

"What's that? Those are cupboards that you, thankfully, cannot get into. Jade, I love you, do you know that?" I grabbed her into my arms, kissed and hugged her, and all the while she was giggling.

Completely taken up with the then-unopened pantry door, Jade asked again, "Wassat?" I put her on the floor and let her continue with her great explorations.

Although it was a warm sunny day, I preferred to stay indoors with Jade. I didn't want to share any of this magic with anyone else. Jade was just incredible, wanting to know what everything was and how it worked. In no time at all, she had lopsidedly inserted a sheet of paper into the typewriter and was gleefully pounding away at the keys. "Play with whatever you like," I said. "What's mine is yours!"

Shortly after supper, I telephoned Joan to advise her of the happy turn of events. She was pleased, as well. "Fine, Gail, I guess we can expect to see Jade on Monday night then."

Sunday was an equally beautiful, warm day. After breakfast, I dressed Jade in a pretty red outfit that had once belonged to my niece, Shannon. Staring at herself in the mirror, Jade smiled with approval. "Pitty," she commented.

"Yes, you do look very pretty, Jade."

With Jade in her stroller, we walked to the corner to wait for a bus. I said, "Can't keep you all to myself forever, Jade. It's time you met your grandparents, cousins, aunts, and uncles."

For someone who normally disliked taking buses, mostly because they took so darned long to come, I certainly enjoyed it today. Jade was standing on my knee while looking out the window. Whenever a passenger boarded the bus, Jade, with an impudent grin, greeted them with a cheerful "Hi!"

I walked into my parents' house, propped Jade onto the kitchen table, and called out, "Surprise, look who's here!" Except for my brother Stephen, who had moved to British Columbia, all of my family was there. Poor Jade, I thought. All these new faces and voices. "She's so cute!" "What a little darling!" "Can I hold her?" "Does she walk yet?" "Do you think she wants some milk?" "Does she like animals?" "Let's show her the dog!" Boy, everyone sure had a lot of catching up to do.

My brother Alan attempted to hold Jade. She cried and held out her arms to me. "Gayo . . . up . . . up!" What a terrific feeling—Jade actually wanted *me* to pick her up.

Alan asked, "Was Jade calling you 'Gail?'"

"Yes," I replied, a little bit defensively. "So what? That's my name. I don't mind her calling me 'Gail.'" *Joan was Mama Joan and I was Mama Gail. That Jade often left out the "Mama" part was not of great importance to me; I'd have gladly gone by any name she'd given me.*

My mother and sisters were already making plans. "Let's take Jade to the zoo, or for a walk by the river, or to Angrignon Park—she'll love to see the seagulls!"

"No," I said, "Jade is with me only for the weekend, and this afternoon, I want to spend as much as time as possible with her—alone. Tomorrow we can bring her to Angrignon Park if you want."

My father didn't say too much. A very reserved, quiet man, he was always difficult to understand, and we never really knew what he was thinking or feeling. My grandmother used to brag about how, when my father was little, he would fall down, and she would scorn him if he so much as shed a single tear. "Brave boys don't cry," she'd say. My father was not one for small talk and appeared to be a little uncomfortable with this new situation. But he did manage a smile.

When my mother questioned me concerning the secrecy of my plans, I explained to her that my whole life had needed sorting out before I could make any commitments to Jade, and I had to do it on my own. I explained, "I didn't want to tell anyone of my plans, until I knew for sure that they were actually going to happen."

Then, in brief detail, I informed my mother about Jade's heart problem, concluding with, "We just have to make sure that Jade does not needlessly tire herself. She doesn't require any

51

medication at this time. So far, so good, and although her colour is generally healthy looking, she tends to get a bluish colouring to her lips and fingernails when she's overly tired. It's called *cyanosis*, and it's also noticeable when she's cold or sick."

After lunch, one of my brothers drove Jade and me back home. Jade took a nap, and we later went for a walk along the boardwalk. She was totally impressed by everything she saw, her eyes lighting up whenever she spotted a baby or child who was about her size. She no longer seemed to be timid among strangers; it was always a friendly, "Hi," and a great big cheerful smile.

We sat down in the grass where we held a serious discussion.

"What do you plan to do when you grow up, Jade?"

Pointing to the river, she answered, "Wassat?"

"That's a river, Jade. Does that mean you are going to be a captain of some large ship?" "Beesje," she answered.

Beesje? What's beesje? I wondered. I knew that a gruffly pronounced *"taw"* meant cookie—more specifically, an arrowroot biscuit—but I was still trying to figure out this other peculiar word.

"Wassat?" Jade asked again, this time pointing to a loose thread on my sweater.

"Oh that's a loose thread that I should fix so I don't end up with a rip, and that would be terrible because I don't like to sew."

"Beesje," she said, this time trying to rummage through the diaper bag to reach for her bottle of milk.

"Beesje. Of course! That means bottle!"

She pulled herself onto my lap, hugged me, then gave me a big wet kiss on the cheek. She climbed back down, pulled some grass from its roots, and asked, "Wassat?" She started to giggle, then threw the grass at me, and I realized that I was being teased.

I grabbed her into my arms and kissed her a hundred times. She giggled some more, threw more grass at me, then started bumming her way toward the concrete pathway.

As planned, on Monday morning I brought Jade to

Angrignon Park, a big green open space, garnished with lots of trees, birds, and squirrels. It was yet another bright, sunny day, and there were many adults, children, dogs, and cyclists. Everyone was out to capture the beauty of this day.

I planned to meet my sisters and my mother at the opposite end of the park from which we had entered. It was about a half hour walk, and every so often I stopped to take Jade from her stroller, pointing out all the things that one sees while on a nature walk.

"Squirrel," I said. "Wowo," she repeated.

"Trees," I continued. "Tees," she said. Then she decided that it was her turn to do the teaching: "Gass, dog, boods, and bikes." And of course, I repeated after her: "Grass, dog, birds, and bikes."

When I met up with everyone, we decided to take Jade to see the seagulls. There was a small man-made lake nearby, a place where the seagulls would most likely look for food. My mother, thoughtfully, remembered to bring a loaf of bread.

We sat in the grass, tearing slices of bread into small pieces, throwing the bits near the lake. Within seconds, a huge flock of seagulls was greedily devouring the food. Jade was so excited. "Wheesh!" she screamed. As Jade sat in the grass, she flung her arms up in the air, demonstrating the seagulls' flying technique. "Wheesh!"

"Yes, Jade, the birds do go wheesh!" It was great fun simply watching her having so much fun. I asked her if she wanted to feed the seagulls, then handed her a piece of bread, which she then threw about two whole feet in front of us. The seagulls were there in a flash, and a worried Jade was yelling, "No, no!" as she scrambled from the scene.

We started to head back home for lunch. As I pushed Jade in her stroller, she started to giggle and pointed to a seagull that was feeding from a nearby garbage receptacle. "Wheesh," she yelled.

When lunch was finished, I placed Jade on the futon so she could nap. I looked at this delightful little person and thought about how lucky I really was. I've truly been blessed in that God gave me such a precious gift. Such an adorable, innocent, affectionate child, who rarely made any complaints. I loved to be there to watch her fall asleep, and I loved to be there to watch her wake up.

> I watch her as she awakens,
> Gently rub her tiny back,
> As she points in three directions,
> With words similar to *What's that?*
>
> She'll want her comforting cuddles
> Until she's fully awake,
> Seems there's so much love to give,
> And so much love to take.
>
> These moments I do cherish
> With all my heart and soul
> And, finally, I've stopped searching
> For I have reached my goal.

I vowed that from then on, every single weekend and holiday, without exception, was to include Jade—my very reason for being.

It felt as though I was a brand new person, just as it had felt on the day Jade was born. Once again, I had that same feeling of contentedness that I'd known after giving birth, that same feeling of exuberance that washed over me as I stood in the soothing warm shower, being reborn.

I worked consistently throughout the week and had more contact with my friends. Absolutely nothing in this world seemed to dampen my spirits. The phrase "Thank God it's Friday," now meant exactly that because, for Jade and me, Fridays were always a new beginning. Directly from work, I'd pick her up from her foster home, then we'd take the subway and bus back to my house or, as I should say, "our" house.

Jade was much more than a daughter. She had become my closest friend. We played together, went out for walks together, sang songs together, and we even danced together. Jade was able to stand, but not without support; I would waltz with her in my arms or, as she sometimes preferred, she would lean against the bookcase, swinging her little arms and swaying her little body to the music. The song entitled, "You've Got a Friend," became *our* song, our waltzing song. And whenever we shared these special times, Jade would touch my face ever so gently, calling me her "fend," then clap her hands when the song was over.

Even though I had Jade on weekends, I nonetheless wanted to participate in her weekly activities as well. Ever since Jade was six months of age, Joan had been bringing her to a learning centre where a stimulation program was offered. The program itself, called "First Step," focused mainly on special education techniques that would stimulate and enhance fine and gross motor skills. This program, geared toward teaching parent and child alike, involved training sessions on how the child could better learn to crawl, walk, grasp fine objects, and so on—all activities of which were set at the individual child's level.

Joan regularly updated me concerning Jade's program and, in turn, I integrated such sessions into our weekend playtime. It was then that I came to realize the extent to which I had taken children's everyday skills for granted. Getting dressed, for instance, required so much more practice for Jade than it would for a "normal" child, as did learning how to form new words, standing without support, walking with support, catching a ball, and so on.

In gross motor skills, Jade was lagging behind by approximately twelve months, but she more than compensated for the delay by means of her fine motor abilities. She had a great concentration span, threaded beads with little effort, held crayons and pencils as would any child her age, and she especially enjoyed piecing puzzles together. Her persistence amazed me. If one single piece didn't fit, she sat there for as long as it took to figure it out and, much to my surprise, she never lost any patience. What's her secret, I wanted to know?

Drawing and scribbling was one of Jade's favourite pastimes. She took a piece of paper and a pencil wherever she went. Each picture had to be acknowledged as a masterpiece, and she made sure that such recognition was granted.

Jade's verbal skills were steadily improving, and Joan and I had certain logical guidelines to follow. The speech pathologist at the Centre reminded us, "One must make talking a fun thing to learn, not a forced thing."

And for Jade, talking *was* a lot of fun. In fact, she never stopped. If she couldn't find an adequate word to express herself, she'd make up her own. I was able to understand most of Jade's words and their meanings, just as she easily comprehended my version. I had to learn *not* to correct, but rather to model a new word by offering it in an exampled phrase. Positive reinforcement was a constant—for both of us!

This coming Christmas was not going to be the sad, dull, lonely Christmas I once knew. This would be my first Christmas with Jade.

Mr. Gibbons often mentioned how much he loved having Jade around, how her laughing and playing was like music to his ears. I thought it would be nice if the three of us could spend Christmas together, but since he already had plans with relatives, Mr. Gibbons was delighted to spend part of the morning with us.

On Christmas day, I woke up earlier than Jade, anticipating the surprise and excitement on her face when she would bum her way into the living room to discover all the gifts.

Finally, at eight o'clock, she woke up.

"Merry Christmas, Jade! I love you!"

"Maymiss-miss, Mama Gayo," she said, wrapping her little arms around me.

After breakfast, Jade went into the living room. "Pesents!" she screamed, "Oh boy, pesents!"

Mr. Gibbons came upstairs to join us. Whenever he came to visit, Jade usually offered him some tea, but not today. She excitedly pointed out the gifts under the tree. "Pesents, Gibbons? Wan some?"

We had so much fun just watching this gleeful little child as she anxiously tore away the wrapping on her gifts.

Mr. Gibbons gave Jade a musical clown, and it was obvious how much she appreciated the gift when she went up to him and planted a big kiss on his cheek, along with a million "Hank you's."

Out of several gifts of clothing, Jade selected the outfit that she wanted to wear to church. Although it was a pretty, velour outfit, I'm sure it was Jade's preference because it came from two of her favourite people, Jim and Joan.

Jade loved going to church, its main attraction being the people. She always anticipated the part of the mass when the parishioners would shake one another's hands and say, "Peace be with you." Jade wasn't the least bit shy and, within the shortest amount of time, made certain to shake as many hands as possible and say, "Piss be you."

Music was another attraction of the church. Jade would pick up the hymn book and sing along, occasionally glancing at me to make sure that I was well aware of her talent. While turning the book right side up for her, I'd whisper, "You're singing beautifully, Jade."

We went to my parents' house later that day and, when dinner was over, Christmas started all over again for Jade. Inundated with gifts, she exclaimed, *"Oh boy! Moe pesents! Awwight!"*

CHAPTER SIX

I was looking forward to the summer holidays. In June, I would take Jade to visit a couple of friends living in Vancouver. It would be her first airplane ride, an experience that I hoped would be memorable.

I pestered Jade to learn exactly what an airplane was. At the airport, as we looked out the window facing the runway, I pointed to a plane that was in full view.

"Airplane," I said. "We are going on a big airplane just like that one."

"Oh, airpane, awwight!" Jade exclaimed.

As we were boarding the aircraft, I again mentioned, "Airplane, Jade. We are now going *on* the airplane."

"Oh yeah?" she said hesitantly.

When we were seated, I said it one last time, "Airplane, Jade. See, *this* is it."

"Yeah, yeah, Gayo—airpane," she replied. I detected a slight annoyance in her voice. Quickly sidetracked, Jade discovered the seat belts, buttons, and trays, all of which had to be tested. She was quite the mechanic.

When Jade spotted the lunch cart, it was as though she had never seen food before. She started laughing and clapping her hands. "Yay! Yay!"

During lunch I just had to say it, just one more time: "What's an airplane, Jade?"

With a sly look upon her face, Jade took her fork, slowly motioning it toward her open mouth, and e-e-e-r-r-r-r- . . . munch! "Airpane," she laughed.

The travelling in itself was probably the nicest part of our vacation. Jade, with her little backpack, was a delightful travel companion. She had a way of bringing laughter to anyone who came her way. She pointed to her glass of milk, looked around at other passengers, and offered, "Mik, mik. My mik, wan some?"

I intervened, "No, Jade, that is your milk. It's very kind of you but you can't offer it to everyone who passes our way."

Jade constantly had to use the bathroom, not because she actually needed to use it, but because it was an excuse to leave her seat in order to greet other passengers and introduce herself: "Hi, me Jade!"

This trip with Jade really was "Flying the Friendly Skies."

When we visited my friends, Jim and Claire, Jade felt right at home. Eager to please them, she instantly won their hearts. She always wanted to know that she was being of some service, either by helping to set the table, feeding the dog, or making up her bed. She was very comfortable sitting for even a couple of hours at a time, just listening and being a participant in our conversations. I couldn't help but be extremely proud of her manners, for Jade seldom interrupted people and she resisted any temptation to touch things that didn't belong to her. She was, in many ways, quite mature.

Like most children, at bedtime Jade decided that she preferred to stay up with the grown-ups. "No tire, me say up, too. Tockin evabody, kay?" She just hated to think that she might be missing out on anything.

During these two weeks we brought Jade on several outings, but she was really missing something—other children to play with.

One afternoon, I was frantically searching for Jade. She had left the backyard and was found "bumming" her way into the street, luckily a cul-de-sac. The neighbourhood children were fascinated and puzzled by her. "Why is she doing that?" they asked. "Look at her go! How can she do that?"

I lifted Jade from the pavement, held her hand, and assisted her to balance as we both walked over to meet the other children. After I introduced Jade to the kids, they showed no interest in playing with her. They just kept staring at her with a puzzled look on their faces. Jade was pulling me back toward the house. She wanted to go back inside. She looked so sad, so humbled. I got the distinct feeling that this was the first time that she had *felt* different. She obviously heard the kids' comments about her bumming around and, perhaps for the first time, she realized she was different.

It just tore me apart to see the hurt in her eyes as she said, "Wanna go home now. Mama Joan's house." And her words were crystal clear.

"Oh, Jade," I said, "I know it's hard sometimes, but guess what?"

She didn't react, just waited for me to continue.

"Tomorrow, we're going to the beach, and we'll have a picnic and go swimming in the ocean, okay?"

"You an me, Gayo?"

"Yes, darling, just you and me. We'll have lots of fun, I promise, okay?"

"Awwight!"

Our vacation to Vancouver had proven too long for Jade, and I looked forward to getting back home, where she was always happy.

In August we were invited to vacation on Prince Edward Island with my mother, my brother, Michael, my sisters, Suzy and Lynn, and Lynn's five-year-old daughter Shannon. It would be a much shorter trip than the Vancouver one, and this holiday would be better geared toward kids.

Shannon and Jade got along wonderfully and it was such a big thrill for Shannon to have Jade look up to her. They adored each other, and Jade imitated just about anything Shannon did or said.

When Shannon was off gallivanting with the others, Jade and I had many private, special excursions of our own. We took glorious nature walks, both of us enjoying the great sense of freedom. Whenever Jade became tired, she requested a piggyback ride. There was something so fresh about life in general: miles of sandy shoreline, the tall grass, the sand dunes, the vast ocean with its roaring waves, and this little kid on my back who was either wanting me to speed up or slow down.

We sat in the grass to rest, and everything was just so interesting. Jade's face lit up; she had such a wonderful smile and intense look.

These moments with Jade were moments of pure astonishment. This was not a fantasy. This was real. And I only had to pinch myself to prove it. Long gone were the days of endless slumber and fantasies, but if I would indulge in one last fantasy, this would be it: Louis Armstrong would be sitting right next to us, singing "What a Wonderful World."

I took this special time to discuss something important with Jade.

"Jade, remember I told you that I'm your mother?"

"No, siddy bum, you Gayo, you Mama Gayo."

"No, Jade, I'm serious; I am your mother. You see, you have two mommies: Joan and me. And you are such a lucky little girl because you have two mommies who both love you very much."

Jade started to giggle, pulled some grass from its roots, then threw it at me. She then grabbed me by the neck, giving me some of her wet kisses, saying, "Me happy, Mommy. You happy too?"

"Yes, Jade. I am very, very happy. You are the best thing that ever happened to me, you know that? "

We returned home from our second trip exactly one day before Jade was to return to foster care, and I to work the day after that. I did the laundry, and Jade helped fold the clothes. Well, she sorted them, anyway. "Diss mine, dat Gayo's, diss mine, dat Gayo's."

I sat down at the kitchen table, feeling sad that our vacation was now over.

"Ah, poe Gayo. Matta?" Jade asked.

I sat Jade on my lap, just needing her cuddles. "Jade,

you're going to Mama Joan's house tomorrow, and I'm going to miss you."

She gently patted me on the back, "Aah, no sad, Gayo. No sad, kay?"

"Okay, Jade, I won't be sad. I love you, and you'll come back next weekend, right?"

"Awwight!"

Jade dashed into the living room to play with some of her long lost toys. She had such an incredible imagination, talking to all of her dolls and trucks, keeping herself amused for as long as two hours at a time, if she so desired. I'm really, really lucky, I thought.

My greatest hope now was that Jade would learn to walk independently. It was becoming increasingly difficult having to accommodate her, this growing child, especially with the heavy winter clothing soon to be worn. While Jade was becoming quite self-sufficient at home, I couldn't very well allow her to crawl up the many stairs in the subway stations. And I couldn't carry her, plus a stroller, plus whatever parcels I might have—it was just too cumbersome and difficult a climb. It often amazed me how some people would observe the struggle, then carry on with their own business, so when someone, usually an elderly person, offered to help, I greatly appreciated it.

I sometimes thought about how much more convenient it would be to have a car. But I couldn't afford the expense and promised myself that I'd avoid debt.

As I'd been doing for some time, I tried to create stimulating situations in order to facilitate Jade's learning to walk. But it became apparent that she also needed to strengthen her leg muscles. I placed her Fisher Price doll house and farm house on a small table in order that she would have to stand while playing with these toys. Then I took two plastic baggies, filled them with sand that I "borrowed" from the playground, inserted the sandbags into a pair of my knee socks, and sewed the ends. As I secured my latest invention to Jade's ankles, she gave me that look, the one that says: "Now you've *really* lost it!" I explained that the weight around her ankles would help build her muscles so she could learn how to walk. She was neither thrilled nor convinced that my theory would work, but with a bit of bribery, agreed to the ankle weights—at least for short periods of time.

I also filled Jade's plastic shopping cart with books, gradually reducing their number as she became more confident with the lighter weight support. But Jade's favourite challenge was when I placed a carpet runner on the living room floor and set it at an angle, so that it made a runway leading to a chair. I perched a large oval mirror on the chair and the coffee table about three feet away. Observing herself in the mirror, Jade would lean against the table, taking a few awkward steps toward the chair. Each time she "made it," she'd laugh nervously and repeat this challenging, yet fun exercise, as I moved the table back an inch or two between turns.

On the evening of October 15, 1982, at thirty-nine and a half months of age, Jade took her first independent steps. Winning a million dollar lottery couldn't have excited me more than seeing the thrilled look on her face as she proudly took baby steps around the house. She kept going from room to room, trying to get used to her new independence.

As I would with any and all of Jade's accomplishments, I grabbed my camera and shot a roll of film. She was ecstatic, wanting more and more pictures taken. She then removed her slippers and tried to put on her shoes. I was so happy that I wasn't about to ask any questions. The answer was soon revealed though, as Jade walked around on the hardwood floors, wanting to hear the sound of her own footsteps. Her walking capability was that of any twelve-month-old who was just starting out. She stumbled a lot, but didn't get discouraged.

On the following Sunday we went to visit my family. Jade especially adored her grandfather, whom she called "Poppa." As soon as we arrived, Jade would quickly walk up to him, grasp her arms around his legs, and give him a big bear hug. She loved to observe Poppa as he sat quietly playing a game of solitaire, which would then turn into a game of double solitaire. I was deeply touched that this feisty little kid had managed to break down her grandfather's strong, silent barrier—a feat nobody, myself included, had ever accomplished before. Something very special had developed between them, and Poppa now meant the world to Jade.

A sports fan, Jade later joined Poppa in the living room. She plunked herself in front of the television, and her little arms flailed around in the air as she cheered and yelled, "Oh no, faw down! Touch Down! Shoots! Scores! Awwite!" It didn't matter what the game or sport was, she liked them all, and because of her sports-minded foster brothers, Jade had opportunities to attend various games where she learned some of the lingo. When our visit was over, Jade would never think of leaving without giving everyone, especially Poppa, a big kiss and a hug. "See ya wetta evabody!"

In December, I explained to Jade that Christmas was a time of giving gifts. "It is Jesus' birthday and, just as you receive presents on your birthday, Jesus wants us to celebrate His birthday by giving gifts to others." Her eyes lit up just as bright as the Christmas tree lights. "Pesents! Awwite!"

Eager to assist with Christmas shopping, Jade was completely taken up with the shopping mall decorations and, of course, the many Santas she had seen. "Cause!" she'd laugh anxiously. "Me see Cause, kay?"

"In a little while, Jade," I assured her. "We need to do some shopping first."

While we were browsing through a book store, with a burst of excitement, Jade exclaimed, "Book Gamma! Book Gamma!" Her whole body was trembling with excitement as she tried to get this obviously important message across. Still pointing to one particular book, she repeated, "Book Gamma!"

"No, Jade," I said, "I don't think we're going to buy that book for Grandma." She sighed and finally gave up.

Then I realized what she had been trying to tell me—that Grandma *has* that book. I was deeply touched by this moment for it meant the world to Jade to be able to communicate clearly enough to have her message understood for its exact meaning. God, what we take for granted! A little child merely wanted to state that she recognized a familiar item yet had so much difficulty in adequately expressing herself. How many "important" messages had I misunderstood or simply brushed aside, I wondered?

Returning home, we waited in the freezing cold for the darned bus to come. As Jade noticed the bus finally approaching from around the bend, she shouted, "Dares it! Take so wong. Wookit. Take so wong."

"Actually, Jade, it's called a *Bus*, not a *Take so long*."

We sat on the long seat at the front of the bus, and seated across from us was a man whom, I suspected, had had a couple of Christmas cheer drinks too many. With no other seating alternative, I was hoping that Jade wouldn't pay too much attention to him, but no such luck. Instantly, they were shouting across to one another. "Boo!" The man started it.

"Boo!" Jade shouted back. "Me Jade!"

They both greeted new passengers boarding the bus. Before long Jade, too, was slurring her words. Whenever the bus came to a halt, both the man and Jade slipped sideways onto the unfortunate person seated next to them. Slightly embarrassed, and trying not to look in too many directions, I just hoped that each coming stop was to be the man's. I could hear all the chuckles, and at a quick glance, I noticed that Jade had attracted a wide audience. Completely aware of this attention, she occasionally turned to me, with a grin of great pleasure.

That Christmas Eve was just as beautiful and magical as any in a movie or storybook. The temperature was very mild, and huge snowflakes fell to the ground.

After dinner I brought Jade outside for a ride in her sled on our way to church. She was absolutely mesmerized by all the colourful Christmas lights and decorations in the neighbourhood, the plywood structures of Santa, his reindeer, and more. She laughed wildly and yelled, "Wookit, Gayo, wookit!" This little child, totally absorbed in every ounce of beauty that surrounded her, truly appreciated more than I would have ever normally recognized.

At 7 P.M., we arrived at the small church just a few short blocks from home. Since Jade loved attending church, I expected that she would especially enjoy participating in a children's mass. I had learned that tonight's mass was to include many Christmas carols and that the children were welcome to participate in setting up the makeshift stable. I remember explaining this to Jade the previous weekend, but just how much she actually understood, I didn't know. In any event, I figured that Jade would observe, as she observed everything else, then take part in the celebration when the confident moment arose.

When the priest invited the children to join him at the altar, Jade looked up at me, awaiting permission. Since she was more confident, and steadier on her feet, when holding my hand, I escorted her to the altar, then returned to my seat in the third pew. Jade joined in the carol singing and, unlike the other children, she applauded and cheered upon completion of each carol.

The children were then requested to set up the stable, adjacent the altar. Jade looked at me, hesitating to join the others. I accompanied her to the stable then returned to my seat once again. She picked up a doll and maternally cradled it in her arms. In a very loud whisper, a shocked little boy, about eight years old, exclaimed, "Hey, don't do that! That's baby Jesus! You're not supposed to hold him! Don't you know that, ya dummy!" He grabbed the doll from Jade's arms and set it back into the cradle.

The boy's mother, seated nearby, came to the rescue. She yanked her son aside and whispered something into his ear. There were about ten or twelve other children there who continued setting up the stable, no longer paying any attention to Jade, the boy, or his mother.

Jade's feelings were obviously hurt, and she helplessly stared over at me, awaiting my rescue. I came over to her and whispered, "Never mind that boy, he's not very nice." She returned with me to our seat and looked humiliated and dejected for the remainder of the mass. When I handed her the carol sheet, she just threw it on the floor, no longer wanting any part of this place.

"Guess what, Jade," I whispered, "When we get home, we're going to make up our very own stable with a baby Jesus, and you can hold Him all you want because He *loves* to be held. Does that sound like a good idea?" With tears in her eyes, she nodded in agreement.

During the latter part of this so-called celebration, all I could think about was that little brat who had belittled my child and called her a dummy. Nobody, at least nobody to my knowledge, had ever called Jade a dummy before. The anger welled up inside of me, and I imagined how satisfying it would have felt to give that kid a good whack across his bratty face. Thank God, mass was over.

CHAPTER SEVEN

In January 1983, Joan had brought Jade to the hospital for her annual cardiology checkup. She reported, "There's been no change—no improvement, but the condition hasn't worsened either." She added, "I don't know how the doctor could hear any heartbeat though, because Jade wouldn't stop screaming or kicking the whole time we were there."

Except at the times of these appointments, I tried very hard to forget that Jade even had a heart problem. But I couldn't entirely forget. There were nights when I would cry myself to sleep. Those nights were reserved for when Jade was not with me. The only thing I could resolve during those worrisome nights was that there was really nothing more I could do, except to love Jade completely and unconditionally. And there was hope—there had to be. Jade was going to stump the entire medical field—she had to. If miracles could and did happen—well, then who more than Jade deserved one?

Nothing made me happier than spending time with Jade. She was always a great burst of sunshine, no matter what kind of week I'd had. I was beginning to resent Sundays, however, for the simple reason that our time together would soon be over. On Sunday evenings, I always had a sad, lost feeling. I'd return Jade to her weekday home in foster care, and then I'd return home—alone. I missed her infectious giggles and the feeling of absolute contentment that came from her hugs and kisses. When she was with me, I'd devour every ounce of her affection, and when she was gone, I'd crave it.

Becoming more and more dissatisfied with this arrangement, I often had to remind myself that because I was a single parent, working full-time, this situation was the most feasible. It was also genuinely clear that Jade truly loved Jim and Joan and their family. She was very happy with them, there were no apparent problems as far as social services were concerned, and Jade was being well-stimulated and well-cared for.

Each time Jade returned to foster care, she was welcomed with open arms by everyone and never showed any hesitation about leaving me. She was so accustomed to this arrangement that I'm sure she had grown to be most comfortable with the loving advantages of both homes. Nevertheless, I still wanted more time with her, and eventually decided that I wanted her full-time home to be with me.

Prior to my taking full responsibility for Jade, I had to be certain that I could make the necessary provisions. After investigating the various day-care centres in and around my own neighbourhood, I learned that a good deal of time would probably be consumed before I could find one that would be suitable. Some centres flatly refused to accept Jade—some without even meeting her. Others would only accept her on the condition that she "fit in" with the group of children, and I was told not to expect anything extra for special needs. In other words, I would have to ignore the fact that Jade would be denied additional help with any gym or play equipment, with learning games, or with *anything*. But I simply couldn't ignore the importance of the extra stimulation time that Jade required.

I wondered if there was a day-care centre, somewhere, whose director would at least try to understand that Jade just required a little more time than the other children did. She needed a little more time to be shown how to do things so that she could follow along with her peers. How else could Jade learn, I politely argued, if not by example?

I continued with my search. I went through the entire telephone directory, limiting the list to centres that were accessible by public transportation, yet close enough to home and work. I realized that finding a neighbourhood day-care centre would be a luxury at that point. If only I could find one that would accept Jade and provide the extra help that she needed . . . I thought of the time when Jade's diagnosis was first explained to me and of the doctor's reassurance: "There will always be help along the way." Well, she forgot to tell me where to find it.

I followed up any recommendations I received. After doing the rounds, I was discouraged to find out that there wasn't a vacant space available or, as it was often put, "Our facility is simply unequipped to take on a handicapped child." Man, I was getting more frustrated by the minute, being turned away time after time, even after I explained, "Jade is just like any other child. She just needs a little extra help, that's all. Surely you don't require any special equipment for that."

Did they not realize, I wondered, that parents of special children needed to earn a living too? Did they think that having a special child gave us special privileges? Did they think that we were exempted from paying rent and utility bills, purchasing clothing and bus passes? Did they think everything in my life was for free?

At this time, Joan asked if I would consider having her baby-sit Jade, as opposed to foster care. While the genuine offer seemed a logical solution, for some reason, I couldn't get past the notion that Jade would still consider my home as secondary and I didn't want to be second anymore. I wanted my home to be the first—the one and the only.

Later, a friend recommended that I enquire at one particular day-care centre, located in Notre Dame de Grace. The large building itself had a very clean, fun atmosphere with lots of educational toys and toddler-sized gym equipment. And at last, I could be thankful that here was a centre whose director was open-minded and willing to give Jade a chance.

A trial period of two weeks was set. This centre, I learned, had already had a positive experience with integrating a child with Down syndrome. I was told that this little girl, named Hannah, was thriving due to the acceptance and friendship of her "normal" peers. Thank you, Hannah, whoever you are! Thank you for opening the door for Jade.

I sublet my flat in Crawford Park, then moved to Montreal West, a small municipality adjacent to Notre Dame de Grace. At this point the move seemed worth the trouble, because I decided that if this particular day care arrangement proved to be unsuitable for Jade, at least we would be living in a more centrally located area where the possibilities of day care would be greater.

In the meantime, Jade's foster mother, who was very supportive of my plans, offered to bring Jade to the day-care centre for short visits in order that Jade might familiarize herself with the setting before the trial period was to begin.

Jade had been exposed to only five or six children at a time at the learning centre, and this new setting created overwhelming insecurities for her. During the first hour of the morning, some seventy-five children were grouped together in one large room. They were later divided into smaller groups of fifteen. Keeping a tight rein on Joan, Jade cried a lot. The noise of the busy crowd frightened her, as did the thought of Joan leaving her for a while.

Having only the very basics of furniture, I took just a couple of days to get completely organized and settled into my new place, a large, older, four-bedroom, upper duplex that I shared with my friend, Jennifer. Shortly thereafter, Jade moved in with us. Jade seemed very comfortable at this new house, but I wasn't too sure whether she realized that this was now her permanent home.

Although Jennifer was not accustomed to having small children around, she and Jade got along fairly well. It turned out to be a very practical and economical arrangement, since Jennifer and I shared the expenses and mutually agreed that Jennifer would not interfere with my raising Jade. There were also other advantages for both of us, such as a barter system. I would tend to a greater share of the household chores, and Jennifer would reciprocate by baby-sitting in the evenings, so I could take some courses at a nearby university.

I planned to keep in close contact with Jade's foster family. Jade and Emmanuel were just like brother and sister, playing with each other, as well as fighting with each other. Their friendship was so special that I wanted it to continue with regular visits.

On Monday morning, I brought Jade to the day-care centre. While I was explaining on the way about how much fun it was going to be, Jade started to giggle nervously, then inquired, "You too, Mommy? You come, too?"

"Yes, darling, I am coming in for a while," I explained, "but I have to go to work today, and I'll pick you up after work."

Well, I never did get to work that day, nor the day after that. Each time I attempted to walk out the front door, I'd look back, and it just broke my heart to see Jade with the saddest, most insecure look on her face. I felt compelled to return to her, wrap my arms around her, and assure her that everything was going to be fine. With tears in her eyes, Jade pleaded, "Say wif me, pe-ease?" And there really was no choice.

On day number three, I thought, this is crazy. Jade knows that I love her and that I would never leave her in a place that I thought to be unsafe. She was just going to have to trust my judgement. I couldn't believe my own courage—I did it! I actually left Jade at the centre and went to work.

Throughout the entire day, I was on the verge of tears. The image of Jade's heartbroken face had been planted in my mind. At lunch hour, I called the centre and was told that Jade hadn't touched her lunch, as often happens with newcomers, and that she was constantly crying for "Mommy."

When I walked into the centre at 5:30 P.M., I saw the group of children sitting in a circle, listening to a story. Jade wasn't with the group. I spotted her sitting alone at a table at the other end of the large room. She was asking for "wawer," but nobody was around to hear her. How long, I wondered, had she been sitting there asking for water?

"Jade," I called out.

"Mommy, oh, Mommy!" she exclaimed.

I went to her, lifted her into my arms, and showered her with kisses. Jade was experiencing such mixed emotion that she was laughing and crying at the same time.

"Did you have a good day?" I asked.

She hesitated, then replied, "Yeah, goo-day. Go home now?" She started to sob.

I held her tighter. "Yes, Jade, We're going home now. We'll come back again tomorrow, okay?" Jade replied, "No, no come back morrow. Say home wif you."

Day number four was a disaster. The moment we got to the entrance of the day-care centre, Jade started to pull away, just as a dog would when brought to the veterinarian's. I assured Jade that I was going to stay a while to meet some of the other children. Most of the kids were in the downstairs playroom, each eating a bowl of cereal. The day-care teacher seemed a very kind, gentle person. She offered Jade some cereal but Jade refused.

There was a piano in this same room. When the teacher began playing, and Jade's attention had been drawn to the music, I decided that this would be the best moment to leave. I said good-bye to Jade and assured her that I'd be back after work. I didn't give her a chance to respond and quickly headed up the stairs. When I reached the top, I waited and listened.

It was a good five minutes before the crying started. I hesitated and waited another five minutes to see whether Jade would calm down, but she didn't. I simply couldn't turn my back. I rushed to comfort Jade, then brought her upstairs with me. We went into the office where I telephoned my boss, Richard. I was so upset that I couldn't speak properly.

"My God, what happened, Gail?" Richard asked. "Has there been an accident or something? Are you okay? Is Jade okay?"

"No, Richard," I replied, choking on the words. "I didn't have an accident. It's worse, I have to leave Jade in day care." Then I started to laugh, but just for a minute. "Jade is in a day-care centre, but I can't leave her here. She's just too unhappy, and she needs me. She needs a mother!"

While I was still talking on the phone, convinced that Jade's world was being torn asunder, she was sitting at the desk beside me, drawing circles and lines on a paper, all the while humming a tune.

Richard was understanding and told me to take the rest of the week off, what was left of it, to work things out and find a solution.

On Friday, I spent the entire day with Jade at the centre, just for one more try. In the end, I recognized that this environment really wasn't suitable. Everything was too busy for Jade, and the noise continued to frighten her. I decided that what she really needed was a smaller, much smaller, setting. It was most unfortunate, I thought, that the one and only day-care centre willing to give her a chance hadn't worked out after all.

Making this decision resulted in a tremendous sense of relief. The guilt had been lifted from my shoulders. There was absolutely no way in which I could possibly force my daughter into a situation that would make her unhappy. Since I was unable to find another day-care centre that served only a small group of children, in all fairness to Jade, she was returned to foster care.

Jade became seriously ill. It was always frightening when she got sick, because there was a constant risk that any illness could cause further deterioration to her heart. And because of her heart condition, Jade wasn't capable of fighting a cold or other virus as easily as most of us could.

This particular virus had developed into pneumonia. Jade was totally listless, had a poor appetite, and slept for most of the three weeks that she was sick. "Please, Lord," I prayed, "please help Jade to get better real soon. I love her so much, and I miss having her with me. Please make her healthy again real soon."

CHAPTER EIGHT

By March, a new social worker, Alice Bigelow, was assigned to our case, and in every sense of the word, she was a worker. She actually listened to real problems and tried to help by finding real solutions. Alice was best recognized amongst her peers, I learned, as a person who was not afraid to bend certain rules or, if required, to take a stand against the government's rigid, single-minded policies when they proved to be useless or unrealistic.

I explained to Alice that all I wanted was to live a normal life with my child, and that I needed help in finding a solution, so that Jade could live with me on a full-time basis. Alice informed me of a "Family Day-Care" program being offered through Social Services. I wondered why Carolyn hadn't told me of this program. There was only one snag, though: the day-care provider, typically a mother at home with children of her own, was not responsible to see that the child concerned was accompanied to and from the learning centre, nor could she be expected to follow up a program at home. Therefore, the stimulation program would have to be discontinued.

I had another important decision to make. Was my having Jade live with me worth her giving up the stimulation program? She'd been a participant since she was six months of age.

Alice was unable to find a provider who was both willing and able to tend to Jade's special needs, but luckily I found a solution. My friend, Karen, who had recently lost her job, was glad to offer some help. She agreed to be the day-care provider at my home. In order to retain my eligibility for a government subsidy, which would help pay the day-care costs, Karen also agreed to work officially under the umbrella of Social Services. At this point, I couldn't have asked for a better friend, or a better solution.

Karen was eager to learn more about children with special needs and enjoyed her involvement at the learning centre. She decided to enrol in evening courses at a local college, in a program called "Techniques of Specialized Education," offered free of charge to (outside) caregivers of children with challenging needs. Why, I wondered, could it not also have been offered to *inside* caregivers, such as mothers? But luckily, after raising a *bit* of fuss, I was also accepted into this program. Not only did I receive a certificate, but my marks also ranked the highest in the class.

By mid-March, we were well on our way to living a "normal" life. It was a great feeling to be able to leave for work in the morning and know that Jade was well cared for in our own home. Karen enjoyed spending time with Jade, and Jade simply adored her.

Leaving work at five o'clock was the best part of the day, for I always anticipated Jade's greeting. Walking from the bus stop to home was a pleasure; every step was one step nearer. When I reached the front door, I was greeted by one delightful little girl who managed to make me feel like the world's most important person. With a big, cheerful smile, Jade would rush over to me, screaming, "Mommy's home! Oh, yeah! Mommy's home!"

In May, I was laid off from my job due to a shortage of work. The layoff was expected to last until late August. In the meantime, I was thoroughly enjoying this uninterrupted time with Jade. I was happy to be able to participate in Jade's program at the centre, and Jade was obviously pleased with my being there. She insisted on showing me around—the different washrooms, the office, the gymnasium, and her classroom. She was proud to point out her works of art displayed on the classroom walls. "Mine," she said. "Did dat seff."

"You did that all by yourself, Jade? Oh, those are the most beautiful paintings I have ever seen! Do you think the

76

teacher will let us take one home?"

In a panic, Jade rushed over to her teacher. "Pichur mine. Take home, kay?"

On the way home, just about every passenger who boarded the bus was stopped by Jade. With a big grin, Jade proudly presented her masterpiece. "Wook! Jade did dat seff. See?"

Jade was just so kissable that I couldn't help myself. Each time I'd observe Jade and her innocent, charming ways, I just had to kiss her.

Trying to look serious, she then squealed: "No, Gayo, top it! Gamma neck, kay?"

"No, Jade, Grandma is not the only one who loves to kiss you on the neck. I'm allowed, too."

Still insisting that it was "Gamma's neck," Jade laughed hysterically as I started to kiss her again.

Jade and I enjoyed a nice relaxing summer, taking long leisurely walks and spending a lot of time at the playground where we built, not castles, but animals, in the sand. The playground sometimes created a little worry, though. One of Jade's favourite activities was the slide. She'd climb up the slide's steps continually and, if I didn't try to stop her, she'd climb until she was out of breath, her lips and nails turning a bluish colour. I'd encourage her to participate in a more relaxing type of activity so as not to exert herself. It deeply bothered me that I had to deny her some of the fun, normal activities that most kids took for granted, but there was a medical fact that just could not be ignored. God, how I hated those reminders.

Absolutely everything we did together was a delight. Even grocery shopping was a fun time for us. Jade would scribble one of her own lists, then search for the items herself. She'd examine the labels, trying to decide whether the item's ingredients were "good" or "no good," or whether its price was "cheap" or "too pensive." Of course people smiled; they couldn't help it.

Jade had an innocent, appealing, often humorous personality. It was amazing how she perceived other people's actions. One day I noticed Jade standing in front of the full-length mirror brushing her hair. When she was finished brushing, she'd turn her back to the mirror, wait for a minute, turn again to face the mirror, and then continue brushing. It occurred to me that Jade had misinterpreted something. She had often observed me brushing my hair. When finished, I'd turn my back to the mirror, glancing to see the back of my head, to make sure I'd done a satisfactory job. Jade just never understood that there was a reason for turning my back to the mirror. Oh well, she got it half right.

Another misinterpretation that I found to be quite amusing was when Jade would flip through a magazine. She'd turn the page using her right hand while simultaneously licking the index finger of her left hand. She never questioned the seemingly odd things people do. Trusting that there was a valid reason, she'd simply imitate an action in the same manner she perceived it. Jade was so trusting of people, in fact, that it sometimes concerned me. I worried that one day somebody was bound to come along, take advantage of her good nature, and thus ruin the pure, loving image she had of this world.

Jade did her very best to try to please others, but not without a lot of frustrating moments. If she couldn't communicate clearly a message to someone, she'd persist until she found the right word to get her point across. If the word couldn't be found, she would act out the message. On one such occasion, Jade wanted Jennifer to give her a board game to play with. Having difficulty in making herself understood, Jade took some coins from her piggybank, set them on the kitchen table, moving each coin while counting, "One, two, fee." When her message became clear, she laughingly said, "Yeah, bo-game, dat's it!" She'd sigh a big sigh of relief while shrugging her shoulders.

Although those frustrating moments were plenty, Jade seldom got angry with anyone, but when she did, she really meant business. Jennifer, almost six feet in height, a smart, self-assured woman, found it hard to believe that this little kid could actually stand up to and reprimand her with a deep, strong voice. "My calator, (calculator) *no* yours. You bad boy, go way, lee me lone!"

Although Jade was quite stubborn at times, she usually gave in to reason, but not without equally interesting recompense, such as playtime on Jennifer's computer. And, just as Jennifer had to refrain from interfering in my raising Jade, I had to refrain from interfering with Jennifer and Jade's battles.

I met my boyfriend, Andrew, during that summer. We met one afternoon while visiting a mutual friend. I don't know if it was the British accent, or the fact that he bore a striking resemblance to a guy I had a crush on in high school, but the attraction was instant. He held an interesting job with an airline, travelled a lot, and had many varied hobbies, mainly in woodworking projects. He seemed down-to-earth with a sense of humour. We talked all afternoon and soon discovered that we had a common interest: a love of nature. Our first date (though we didn't call it that) was a hike in the woods the following morning while our friend, Richard, baby-sat Jade.

We later picked up pizza to bring back to Richard's. Jade kept herself amused playing with her Barbie dolls all afternoon, and every so often, she'd come over to ask Andrew to help her change one of the doll's outfits. Andrew obliged and was very friendly with her.

It seemed odd that Andrew never asked me about Jade. Was it possible that he didn't even notice she was different? If he did notice anything unusual about her, he never let on. I was surprised when he asked me out to a movie. This was really strange, I thought. By now he already knew I was a single mom with plenty of commitments and responsibilities, and yet he asked me out anyway.

After the movie, we talked nonstop as we meandered the cobblestone streets of Old Montreal. Later, over drinks at one of the small bistros, I suddenly didn't have anything to say. I just kept thinking that I really liked this guy, but what were our chances once he found out about Jade, about her special needs, and about what that meant in terms of how much time I had available for anyone else? Knowing this could well be our last date, I nonetheless had to be up-front, and I was. "My daughter has Down syndrome; I just wanted you to know that."

"Yeah, I know," he said. And that was it. No questions asked. No "Well, gotta run; it's been nice . . ."

Our relationship flourished; Andrew treated me with such kindness. At first, Jade didn't approve of my having a boyfriend. She felt threatened, as she wasn't used to sharing me. "My Gayo," she'd remind Andrew, "No you Gayo!" When Andrew and I sat on the sofa, Jade kept a close eye on him. She was like my bodyguard. Sometimes she would go off to her room to play but returned often to check on us and, at one time, caught us kissing. Andrew then swiftly removed his arm from my shoulder, saving Jade the bother of doing it herself.

On the positive side, having a guardian, plus a roommate, was perhaps a good thing. With the lack of privacy, Andrew and I weren't likely to become more intimate anytime soon, which was just as well, since I needed more time. I needed to learn how to trust again and needed to feel loved for who I was. It was important to me that our first time, and every time, be special.

I was recalled to work in early September, but Karen, my God-sent baby-sitter, had since found other employment. Knowing my job was now in jeopardy, I quickly sought other options, such as a preschool program that also offered day care as an extra.

I went through the usual routine. There was nothing available, as each place referred me to another for a possible "better" service.

Trying to avoid the only other option of foster care, I decided that it would be best to enrol Jade in a stimulation program at a centre situated much closer to home than the last centre. And, from here on, my new task was to unravel an endless string of bureaucratic red tape.

Funding for the special bus service could not be provided without a complete breakdown of my expenses, written reports explaining why it was necessary for Jade to attend a learning centre, etcetera, etcetera, etcetera. Jade attended the learning centre anyway, and months later, the funding finally came. It was a nominal sum of money—hardly worth the effort of providing the government with our entire life history.

In November I received a progress report on Jade from the educators at the learning centre. She was a very high functioning child, as I could have told them from the beginning, but the report also stated that she was lacking in social skills. She was somewhat withdrawn and only played independently. This certainly did not sound like the Jade I knew, who was a very sociable child, known to participate in anything and everything.

Once happy to go to "school," as she preferred to call it, Jade was now becoming very upset every morning and refusing to leave the house. One morning, while I was preparing her lunch for school, she went into my bedroom, stripped off her clothing and got into bed. The bus arrived, and I called out to her. No reply.

While the driver was impatiently honking his horn, I found Jade in my bed, comfortably snuggled up in the covers. "No coo day, Mommy. I sick."

"Jade, the bus is here now. You have to go to school." I removed the covers from her, saw that she was naked, then ran downstairs to inform the driver that Jade would be absent that day.

I returned to Jade. She was no longer in my bedroom. She was no longer sick either. Sitting on her little wicker chair about two feet away from the television, Jade exclaimed, "Wook, Mommy, Sessmee Tweet!"

"Okay, Jade, you can watch *Sesame Street*," I said, as I dragged the chair back a few feet with her still in it. "But are you sure you're not too sick to watch television?"

"No, I betta now," she replied with a slight, mischievous grin.

I arranged a meeting with Jade's educator, Lorraine. She

advised me that the centre's student ratio was growing and that the group now included many children with behavioural problems. "At times, these kids take some of their frustration out on Jade," she said. "I think they know that she is not going to fight back and, therefore, she's an easy target. Because Jade is a gentle, unaggressive child, she becomes very sensitive and insecure, thereby withdrawing from many group activities."

"This is all beginning to make sense now," I responded. "Why wasn't I told of this problem sooner?"

"Well," Lorraine answered, "we are doing our best to resolve the problems with some of these kids."

I told Lorraine about how this environment was affecting Jade at home: her refusal to go to school and her newly learned aggression when she returned home afterwards. "Jade sometimes comes home from school," I explained, "takes her favourite doll and behaves aggressively toward it. She grabs the doll by the hair, hits it in the face, then throws it across the room, yelling, *Bad boy, Jo-Jo*! But what I especially don't understand is that this doll is a very special doll to Jade. Her sudden change in behaviour really worries me."

"Well," Lorraine said, "we have two children at the centre who, for no apparent reason, like to bite other kids. We have requested the intervention of a psychologist, who has advised us to separate the child concerned from the others as a form of punishment, or if that doesn't work, we try to encourage the child to be affectionate with the others."

In an angry tone of voice, I asked, "Do you honestly expect Jade to be receptive to affection from a kid who is normally so aggressive?" I then added, "Has Jade ever been bitten?" Now I was trying hard to recall if I ever noticed any suspicious marks on Jade.

"No, she hasn't," Lorraine replied. "She gets pushed around a little by certain kids, but I am constantly encouraging her to push back. She needs to learn how to stand up for herself. As soon as Jade sees those particular children heading her way, she scurries off to the other end of the room. So she can avoid them, she makes herself constantly aware of where these children are at all times."

"What is she learning?" I asked.

Lorraine answered, "During the hour of free-play, as I told you, Jade is unsociable. But during a more structured time, when we are seated at our tables, she is very interested in whatever we are doing. She enjoys fitting puzzle pieces together; she loves to paint and colour, to mould different shapes out of play dough, and to string beads. And she follows just about everything she is instructed to do. Jade has, in my opinion, excellent cognitive and fine motor skills. Her gross motor skills require a lot more work, though. Right now we are trying to teach her how to jump."

Since my meeting with Lorraine, I planned to more closely monitor Jade's reaction toward school. She usually anticipated going to school on Mondays, after the weekend break, but by Tuesday, it started again: "No coo, Mommy. I sick."

Taking Jade's reactions and feelings into serious consideration, I figured it should mostly be her own choice as to when she wanted to go to school, and she chose to attend every other school day. Fortunately, my employer allowed me to work flexible hours during this time.

One day, Jade came home in an unusually quiet mood. Heading directly to her bedroom, she didn't say a word to me. She sat on the floor and started to sob. I went to comfort her and put my arm around her trembling little body. "What happened?" I asked. "Did something bad happen at school today?"

"No coo, Mommy. No more coo, kay?"

Jade buried her head in my lap and continued to sob. As I was about to lift her into my arms, she cried, "Omm hutts." I rolled up the long sleeves on her shirt but hadn't noticed anything unusual. "Omm hutts!" she insisted.

I carefully removed her shirt and noticed teeth marks on her right shoulder, cutting right through the skin. "Oh, Jade, from now on you can stay home with me, okay?"

I promptly checked Jade's health records to determine whether her tetanus shot was up to date. I decided right then and there that I would cut back my work hours to part-time and hire a baby-sitter to fill in those hours. No more luxuries, I decided. I would simply cut out any special treats or desserts I occasionally bought at the grocery store, the monthly bottle of wine I liked to share with friends, and the occasional taxi expenses we'd incur when the weather was bad. I would walk or cycle more in order to eliminate the monthly bus pass expense, and I would simply cut out anything that wasn't absolutely necessary. In this way, I could probably manage to afford working on a part-time basis.

I telephoned Lorraine at the centre. She claimed that nothing unusual had happened that morning. After further thought, she said, "Jade not only refused to participate in the free-play activities, but she also refused to participate in the arts and crafts class." She continued, "I thought that Jade might have been a bit tired because she laid herself down on the gym mat about a half hour after arrival and wanted to remain there until the end of the session."

Trying to keep my cool, I asked, "Do you want to know why Jade was lying on the mat all that time? It's because some kid stuck his teeth into her shoulder, that's why! I'm sorry," I went on, "but Jade will not be returning to the centre, at least not until the problem kids can be controlled. And do you know what? Do you know what Jade is really learning at your centre? She's learning to hate school, to be afraid of other kids, and to be aggressive. That's what she's learning!"

Lorraine came to visit us at home the following afternoon. We discussed more fully the problems that had arisen at the centre. I mentioned that I felt that the stimulation program, at this time, was doing more harm than good. Lorraine confided: "Between you and me, if Jade were my child, I would strongly consider a regular day-care facility where there are "normal" children Jade can model from. You see, at the centre, Jade is the highest functioning child. As you know, most of the children in the program have severe, multiple handicaps. While there are children who can model from Jade, there isn't another child that Jade can model from in a positive way."

She continued, "We have such a wide variety of problems and very little in the way of government funding. It would of course be more beneficial to all of our children if their problems could be dealt with individually. The centre has made numerous requests for extra funding so we could hire additional staff, regroup the children into smaller groups—thereby having a smaller student-teacher ratio—but the government just hasn't come through."

When Lorraine left, I gave her advice some very serious thought. And she was right. Children learn from other children. But at that point, I didn't even know if I could consider a day-care or preschool program, should I in fact be lucky enough to find one willing to accept Jade. I worried that she might have lost *all* trust in *all* children. If she was approached by another child, even a familiar neighbourhood child, she would scurry toward me, grab onto my leg, and lead me to the house for security.

It became an absolute priority for me to help Jade rebuild her trust in other children. I felt so damned guilty and angry with myself that this had to happen at all. Things had been running so smoothly for Jade up until the time that I had decided to have her live with me.

Jade's progress was evaluated by a team of specialists at an assessment and guidance clinic. The team, which consisted of a psychologist, physiotherapist, nurse, and special education teacher, mutually agreed that Jade had acquired very good cognitive and fine motor skills, and they strongly recommended that she receive preschool stimulation. Easier said than done. The team also agreed that Jade's gross motor skills required greater stimulation. They suggested that I look into a swimming therapy program that might be available within the various communities.

After many inquiries, I found a community pool that offered a swimming therapy program. After taking my part-time salary into consideration, however, I determined that I simply couldn't afford it. I applied for funds from Social Services, but my application was denied, and Jade was therefore denied enrolment in the swimming program.

I was delighted to learn of a small "Home Day Care" soon to open within our vicinity. It was run by a woman named Andrea Biondi, who had several years of child care experience and a degree in early childhood education; it was Andrea's intent to set up an educational, child-care service in her own home.

Andrea was willing and fully capable, she assured me, of running a structured, educational program for approximately eight to ten children. Perfect, I thought. Just what Jade needed—a homey environment with a small number of children. But the only problem was that this was private day care, not subsidized by the government. In any event, I had been assured in the past by Social Services that support would be available, should I require it, and again, I applied for funds.

Andrea was very understanding of Jade's special needs and was willing to help in every way possible. She was pleased to learn, though, that Jade didn't really require that much more time than any of the other children. Jade dressed herself with little assistance when getting ready for an outing; it only took a little while longer to walk to the library, and sometimes an additional, more simplified explanation was required to relay a message to her.

In a short time, like the other children, Jade succeeded in learning to do a somersault. She became the main initiator of all games, the others happily joining in. It was a good feeling of accomplishment to see this delightful little child who was now participating in all activities, and on our journey home, Jade spoke fondly of her "fends." The only complaint she had now was that day care was closed on Saturdays and Sundays. Come Monday, though, there was one eager little girl rushing around to get ready for school.

I had contacted Alice at Social Services to follow up my request for financial assistance for the Day Care/Nursery School Program. I was informed, however, that because the day care program in which Jade was enrolled was not a service being offered under the umbrella of the government's Social Services, financial aid would not be granted. But Alice understood my reasons for choosing this particular small day care setting and assured me that she would investigate other funding possibilities.

Several weeks went by before I heard from her again. I always made a point of setting aside a small amount of money from each paycheque as an emergency fund, but by now, my savings account was nearing depletion. With only a part-time salary, I was anxious to learn whether or not I could continue with this program for Jade. Alice was extremely disappointed to tell me that no funds were available.

"Alice, I don't understand this," I said. "Why was I told when Jade was born that there were support services to help lessen the so-called burden of having a child with special needs? The only freaking burden I have is in trying to obtain these services!"

"Gail, I'm really sorry," Alice replied. "I'm doing everything I can, sitting through meeting after meeting, writing memos, and trying my best to explain your situation to my supervisors. I'm going to continue to fight on this issue, and it might be a good idea if you would personally write to Social Services."

"Why is it that Joan never ran into these problems?" I asked. "What if Jade were still in foster care, what then? As a foster mother, would the funds be available to her?"

Alice responded, "I know it doesn't make any sense, Gail, but yes. There are funds available to foster parents who are interested in enrolling their foster child in any program intended to enhance the child's potential."

"Then could it not be explained to whomever is in charge of funding that Jade is not in a day-care centre for the usual reasons? I am living on a part-time salary, not out of laziness, but because the government won't provide me with any alternatives, other than Welfare Assistance, which I will never resort to, or placing Jade into the foster care system. And now, all I'm asking for is some assistance to keep Jade in a program that is remarkably improving her self-esteem, social skills, language, and gross and fine motor skills."

I then wrote a letter to the Director General of Social Services, hoping to convince him of the unfairness toward us and, hopefully, to bring about a policy review.

I waited anxiously for the reply. I knew for sure that Social Services would have to understand my frustrations and make allowances under the circumstances.

The reply came in the form of memorandums that included input from the various social service departments. After reading the memorandums, I felt that I had raised an important issue regarding children with special needs living in their own family. It was indeed the case that special needs children in foster care often received more services than children in their own homes.

This had truly been one hectic and frustrating year. I loved my daughter immensely, but acquiring services for her was like getting blood from a stone. Over the next year, I exchanged a number of letters with Social Services on the issue of enhanced support, and they held several meetings—but without any results. The last I heard in this regard was that the Director of Social Services had *assumed* that Jade was returned to foster care in order to receive support services. Case closed. While it was a battle worth fighting, I no longer had the energy or patience to pursue the matter any further.

On the first of May, due to her own financial constraints, Andrea was forced to close her day-care centre. It was a very difficult time for Jade, because no matter how much I tried to explain to her, she still couldn't understand why she couldn't return to school. I didn't dare seek other options for the time being. I felt confident that after Jade's positive experience at Andrea's, she would adapt easily to summer day camp, which would be starting up soon.

CHAPTER NINE

Because Jennifer had plans to move in with her boyfriend, and I couldn't afford the upkeep of the large flat on my own, I decided to move as well. Jade spent the weekend with Jim and Joan, and with my brother's help, I moved to another nearby duplex that was smaller and less expensive.

The move was not a big deal to Jade. When she came home on Sunday night, she wandered around the house, inspecting each of the five small rooms and all of the closets and cupboards. "Nice," she said, as she continued with the inspection, making certain that all was in place as it was in our former home. She approved of her bedroom and made only minor changes, such as the arrangement of the items on her desk.

Jade was accepted into the neighbourhood day camp. The camp counsellor, Mary, was a bright, friendly teenager with an extremely outgoing personality. She expressed herself lovingly and clearly, making each child feel of great importance. Jade simply adored her and she *loved* going to camp.

Jade was so proud and excited when she was given the camp's blue T-shirt, for it was identical to the one worn by all the other kids. An excellent policy, I thought, for it would help Jade feel that she really did belong. Another thing that made her feel more comfortable was the fact that, being smaller in size and less mature than a typical child her age, she was placed with a group of children who were one year younger.

Jade enjoyed all the camp activities: the songs, the games, swimming, bus outings, and especially the song that the campers would sing on the public bus, no doubt piercing the other passengers' ears.

Whenever Jade and I went somewhere by bus, she now insisted that we sing that same song: "The wheels on the bus go round 'n round . . ."

Because of Jade's heart problem, she tired easily. I asked Mary whether she and Miranda, the counsellor-in-training, were being presented with any difficulties.

"Oh, it's not really a problem," Mary said. "Usually when our group is on an outing, if Jade gets tired of walking, she just plunks herself down on the sidewalk, and then the whole group sits down as well. If we are pressed for time, either Miranda or myself simply give Jade a piggyback ride. Jade is very special to us."

The words "thank you" just didn't seem like enough. I was so grateful that these two teenagers were so compassionate and understanding.

Whenever I met Jade at the campsite, I made a point of arriving a few minutes early. It was the most wonderful feeling in the world to see Jade as "one of the gang," and accepted as such. For Jade and me, normality wasn't something that could be taken for granted, because any new experience for Jade usually required a trial period. But this was great—I had been able to enrol Jade in a community program, without any conditions whatsoever being set.

One day, Jade noticed me waiting for her by the fence. In a burst of excitement, she quickly grabbed her lunch box, screaming, "Mommy's here! Mommy's here!" Trying to rush, she stumbled to the ground, and the lunch box went flying through the air. She got up again, screaming, "Mommy's here!"

She leaped into my arms, smothering me with dozens of hugs and kisses. "Fun, Mommy! Day camp fun!"

When we arrived home, Jade darted into her bedroom, grabbed Jo-Jo, and showed the doll how to play a new game. Once Jo-Jo had apparently learned the rules of the game, my participation was requested as well. We must have played "duck-duck-goose" and "tisket-tasket" a hundred times that afternoon.

There were so many interesting activities at day camp that

Jade didn't have a chance to get bored. On dress-up day, she spent a good half hour in front of the mirror, making sure that her pirate costume was exactly right. When given the opportunity, she loved to experiment with Halloween makeup. When she finished decorating her own face, Jade then experimented on her dolls.

Then there was "Competition Day" at camp. I was feeling so uneasy about it that I procrastinated about whether or not to send Jade that day. I worried about her feelings. She couldn't really run, but rather she'd just hasten her walk. Even then, if she walked too quickly, she'd most often stumble to the ground. She wasn't capable of jumping, for she couldn't manage to lift both feet from the ground simultaneously, and she couldn't catch a ball unless it was being thrown from a maximum three-foot distance.

Still tormented about whether to consent to her participation in this event, I finally determined that this is the real world, and I should not deny Jade opportunities, even if it meant opportunities to fail. She deserved to learn how to compete like everyone else.

After I left Jade at the campsite, I went home to tidy the house and do the laundry. What should have been a simple task proved difficult, as my thoughts were preoccupied with the morning's events. My poor baby, she is going to be heartbroken; she is going to be ridiculed. Please, God, let her win at something!

When I returned to camp to meet Jade, I was more or less expecting to find a tearful, hurt little girl in need of a lot of consolation and cuddles. Instead, I saw one ecstatic kid who was proudly yelling, "I a winno! I a winno!"

She had so many ribbons that they were slipping out of her tiny hands. As Jade bent down to pick one up, another would fall to the ground.

"Wook, Mommy. I a winno! I a winno!"

I was so happy that I just wanted to jump up and scream. "Jade, I'm so proud of you. You must have had a lot of fun!"

"Oh, yeah," she replied, "I a winno, Mommy, I a winno."

"You sure are a winner, darling. And I love you."

I went over to see Mary. Still uncertain how all these winnings could have happened, I enquired, "How did Jade win all these ribbons?"

Mary laughingly said, "Just read the small cards stapled to the back of each ribbon. Jade was terrific!"

Jade handed me the ribbons, pointing out the cards, saying, "Wookit, Mommy, weed dem."

I read them: "Second Place in the Frisbee Throw," "First Place for Walking in Water," "Fifth Place in the Popsicle Hunt," "Fourth Place for Kicking the Ball," and "Third Place for Catching the Balloon."

I felt like a fool and couldn't stop laughing. Why I was expecting something like the International Olympics, I'll never know.

"Jade, because you were so terrific in the competition, I have a special surprise for you. Would you like to go to a movie on Saturday?"

"Satday? A movie? Awwite!"

The ribbons never left Jade's sight for a moment. She put them in a large, blue tote bag, which, over the next few days, went everywhere with her. And at nighttime, Jade placed the bag alongside her pillow.

As promised, I brought Jade to see the movie, "The Wacky World of Mother Goose." Before entering the cinema, we first stopped off at a convenience store to buy some treats—much cheaper than buying at the cinema.

It was Jade's first movie at a cinema, and I was just as excited as she about the new experience. I loved to watch her, because her reactions were always so amusing.

Weighing only thirty-two pounds, Jade just couldn't get comfortable in her seat. It kept flipping upwards, leaving her in an awkward sitting position, her legs being lifted parallel to her head. Consequently, throughout the film, I kept my hand on her seat as an extra weight to prevent it from flipping.

Jade didn't watch much of the film; she was more interested in watching the people around her. She often glanced at me and, with a grin, offered, "Some chips, Mommy? Wan some?" She then continued to look around, commenting, "Many chairs, eh? Many chairs."

"Yes, Jade, there are many seats in the theatre because there are usually a lot of people who come to watch a movie. Aren't you going to watch it?"

"No, Gayo, you siddy. I eat chips. You watchin movie, kay?"

Jade made many new acquaintances that summer. When we went out for a walk, or to do the groceries, she'd greet numerous people—calling them by name. I was impressed but also curious, because half of these people I didn't even know. As I soon found out, most of the people in the community knew Jade. It was always, "Hello, Jade. How are you today?"

"I fine hanks," she'd reply.

Jade would then point to me, making her introductions: "My mommy—Gayo."

Because of Jade's friendliness, I too met a lot of people, some of whom became good friends.

I was always pleased when Michele, our twelve-year-old neighbour, came over to visit. She and Jade got along well. With Jade's plastic bat and ball, they'd play baseball in the backyard. Michele was very patient and enjoyed keeping Jade amused and, much to my relief, Jade got plenty of chances to play her duck-duck-goose games.

Gregory, our downstairs neighbour, often came up to visit. Just a year older than Jade, Gregory was a perfect playmate. He always said that Jade had neat things to play with: lots of paints, crayons, play dough, puzzles, games, books, playing cards, a flute recorder, a musical organ, a tape player, and lots of dolls and trucks. With all of these neat things, though, Jade and Gregory would usually end up lying on the bedroom floor, drawing pictures and colouring them in. Both kids were very creative, proudly displaying their works of art in the art gallery—all the walls in the building's stairwell.

One afternoon, Gregory came running into the kitchen to show me something. He held up one of Jade's cue cards, saying,

"This word says 'School,' right?" "Yes, that's right," I replied.

He exclaimed, "Oh my gosh, I don't believe it!" He then held up another card, asking, "What's this word?"

"That word is 'Emmanuel,'" I answered. "Jade has a friend named Emmanuel, and she wanted to know what his name looked like in print."

"Oh, my gosh!" Gregory exclaimed again. "When I asked Jade what these words were, she got them right! I don't believe it!"

Gregory ran into the bedroom, yelling, "Jade, I've got some more cards for you to read, okay?"

As if making a dare, Jade said, "Okay, moe woods, gimme moe woods."

We celebrated Jade's fifth birthday at my parents' house. It was a beautiful sunny afternoon, perfect for an outdoor party. I filled Jade's plastic swimming pool with water and lots of colourful balloons. Andrew, my parents, brothers and sisters, and I spent the afternoon in the yard with Jade. She loved the attention—so many people taking turns to play games with her—and she especially loved to play with her new ball and plastic tennis rackets.

During game intermissions, Jade leaped in and out of the pool, throwing the balloons into the air, then trying to catch them before they landed in the water. What joy she captured! And what joy I captured in watching this vivacious little child, with her squeals of delight and wonderful happy smile.

Jade's eyes lit up when she saw the big chocolate layer cake coming her way. She got so excited that she had to stop, take a breath, then laugh again. When we finished singing "Happy Birthday," Jade clapped her hands, cheering, "Hooway, I *five* taday!" She then spotted her aunt Suzy coming out from the kitchen carrying an armful of gifts. She exploded, "Pesents! Booday pesents! Oh God!"

Jade anxiously looked around the yard, wanting to make

sure that Poppa was nearby to share in this thrilling event. It didn't take much to please Jade, and I'm sure that had she received but one simple gift, she would have been just as happy.

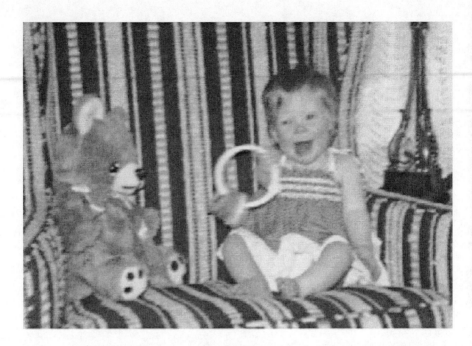

1st Birthday

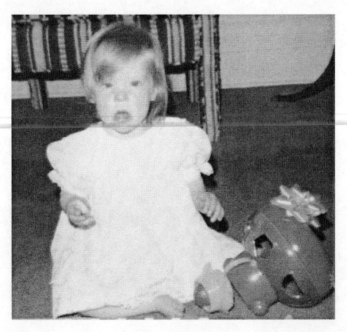

2nd Birthday

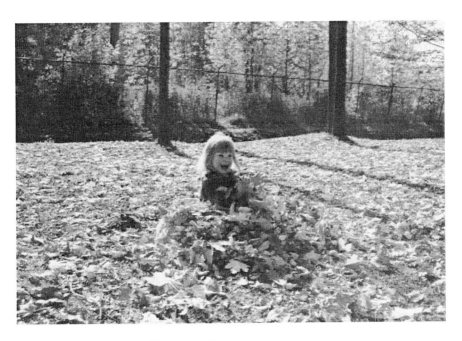

Enjoying the autumn leaves

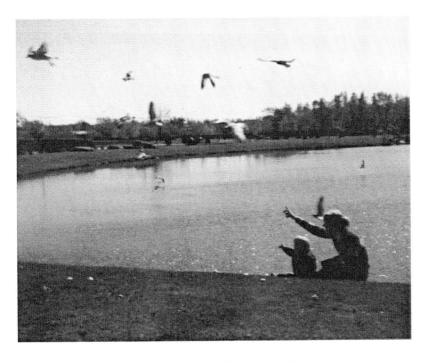

Observing the "wheeshes"

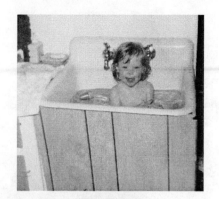

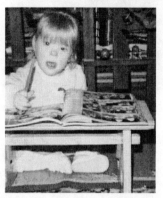

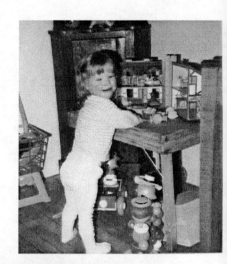

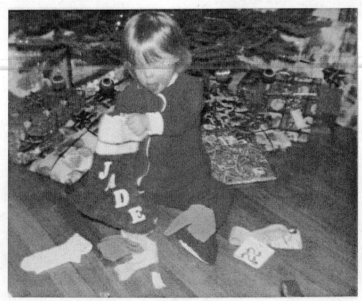

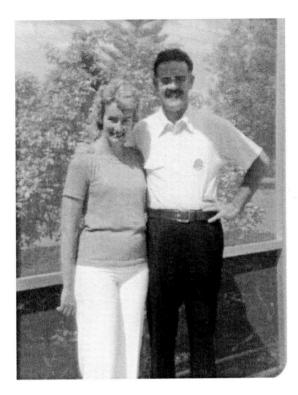

Foster parents, Jim and Joan

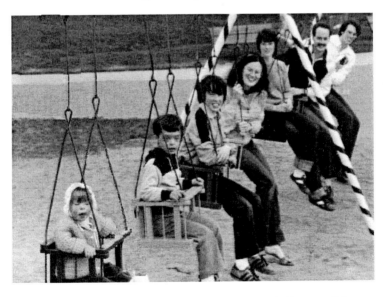

Jade with foster brothers and sisters: Emmanuel, Danny, Margaret,
Anmarie, Myles and Lorne

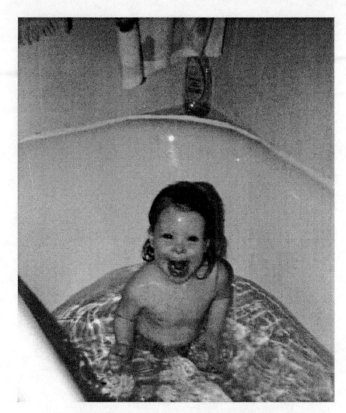

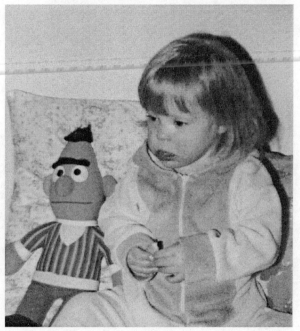

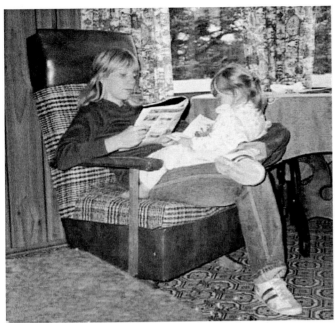
Jade and Gail: downtime

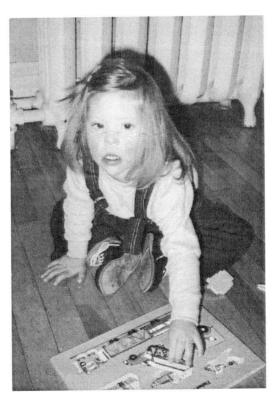

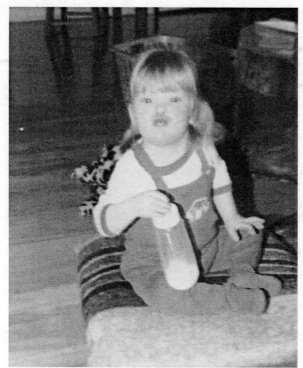

A kiss for . . .

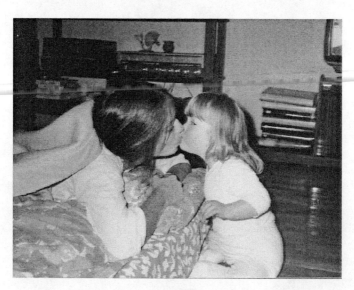

Karen

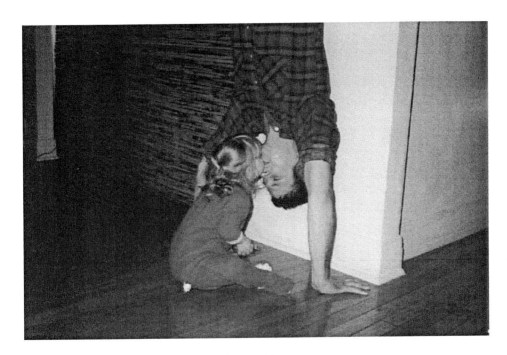

uncle David

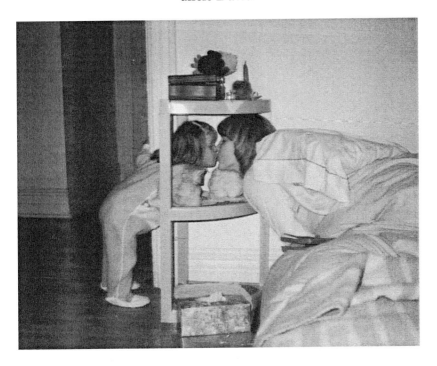

Jennifer

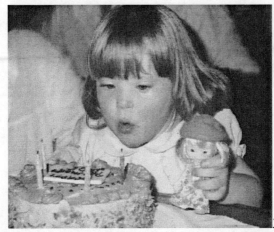

3rd Birthday

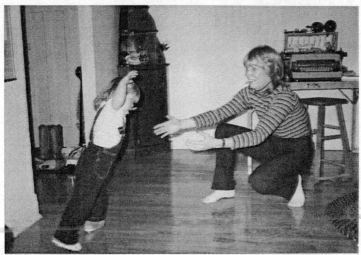

Milestones

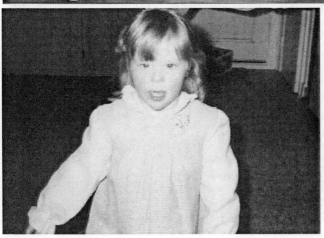

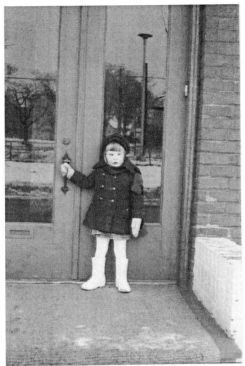

Off to Preschool

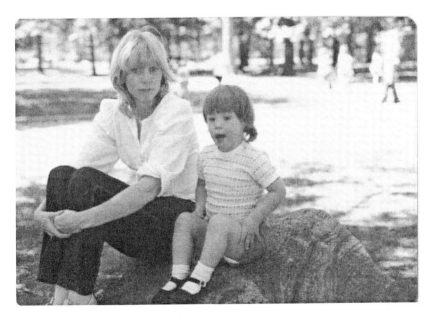

Jade and Gail

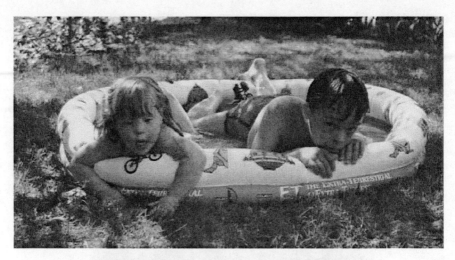

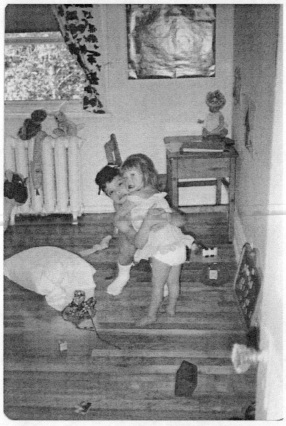

Jade and Emmanuel

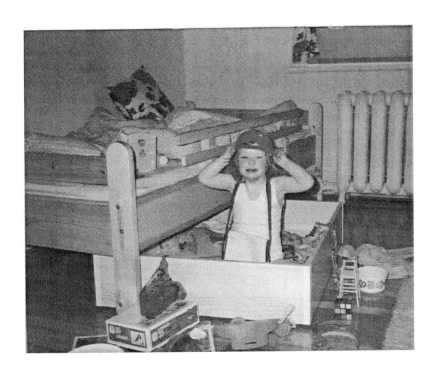

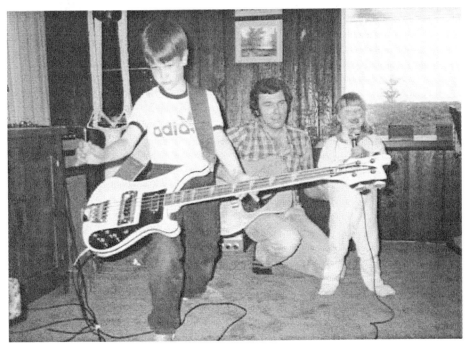

Belting out a tune with Andrew and cousin Michael

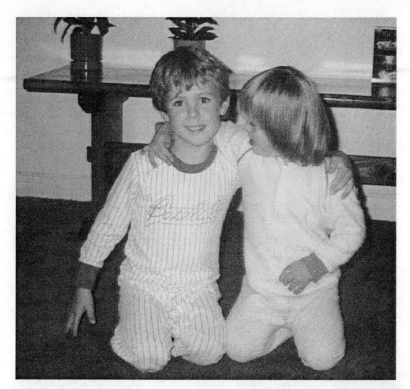

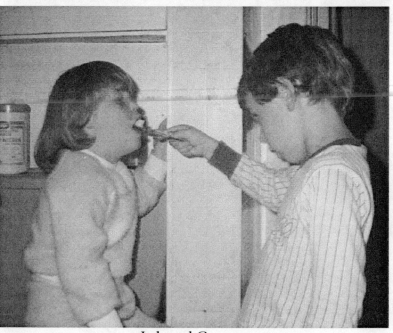

Jade and Gregory

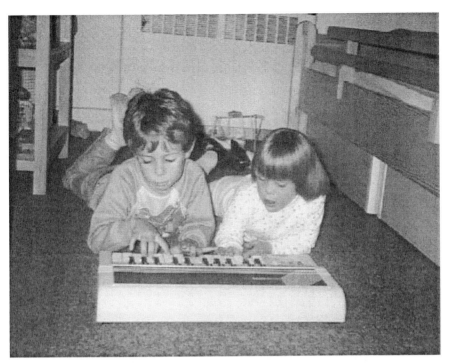

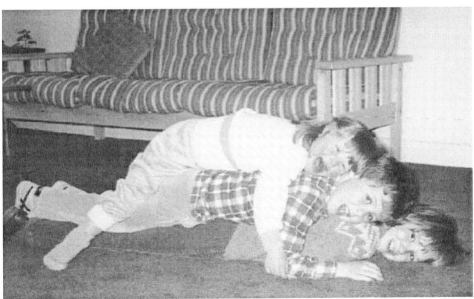

Fun with friends

CHAPTER TEN

In September Jade started school. It was a school that specialized in educating students who had various developmental disabilities. In a previous meeting, the school's principal had assured me that Jade would be provided with a good education. The principal strongly emphasized the fact that the school employed highly qualified special education teachers, a social worker, nurse, speech pathologist, and physiotherapist. Jade's class had an eight-to-two ratio of students to staff. In addition to the special education teacher, there was also a teacher's assistant.

With all of these positive notes in mind, I was still somewhat apprehensive about sending Jade to a segregated school. Although the school, situated in the north end of town, provided a bus service, it nevertheless required two hours per day of travelling time for Jade. At only five years of age, Jade spent most of her day at school: four hours in class and another two hours in commuting. It wasn't so much the distance that made it a long journey but the numerous rounds the driver had to make.

The more I thought about it, the more I hated the fact that Jade had to be sent off to some faraway school. What about her friends? She would no longer see the neighbourhood kids on a regular basis, nor would she be able to share her school experiences with them. How then was Jade ever going to establish and maintain any friendships?

Jade seemed to adapt to her new school. I kept in close contact with her teacher by means of a daily communication booklet that Jade brought to and from class.

With Jade gone most of the day, I increased my work

hours but ensured that I arrived home before she did. When the bus driver, Gary, pulled up at the front of the house, I'd rush out to greet Jade. Often she'd be in a sound sleep and Gary would say, "Wake up, Jade. You're home now. Wake up, you sleepyhead." Gary then said, "All I know is that she must be really tired to be able to sleep on this bus with all the noisy, screaming kids." The kids on the bus were of all ages, ranging from four to eighteen years old. Poor Jade, I thought, such a big day for someone so little.

Jade followed me into the kitchen and sat down at the table to keep me company while I prepared supper. "How was your day at school, Jade?"

"Fine," she replied. She started to peel a banana, then added, "Wanna fammy."

"You want a fammy? I don't understand, Jade, what's a fammy?"

"Budders, sissers, daddy," she answered.

Taken aback, I said, "Oh, you want a family! Jade, we are a family. You and me."

"Jade daddy?" she inquired.

"Oh, sweetheart," I replied, "your father lives someplace else and there's nothing I can do about it. But Jim is like a father to you, and you love him, don't you? And Andrew is good to you and he loves you. And guess what? You do have a big family. You have a grandmother, a grandfather, four uncles, three aunts, and two cousins. So, you see, we do have a big family."

I didn't know what else to say. Seeing the disappointment in her eyes and listening to the sadness in her voice, I just wished that I could have snapped my fingers and had an instant family, the kind of family that Jade was now asking for—one that included a daddy and a brother and a sister.

Without saying a word, Jade wandered off into the living room and turned on the television while I went downstairs to get the laundry out of the basement. A few minutes later, she was back in the kitchen with a big, black cat dangling from her arms.

"Where did you get that?" I asked. She shrugged her shoulders, then pointed to the back door.

97

"Oh, he was waiting at the door?"

Jade shook her head, then sat on the floor to pet the cat. "Ah, cat's cute, eh, Mommy. I keep it, kay?"

"No, Jade. I know this will be hard for you to understand, but I'm allergic to cats. They make me itchy, and they make me sneeze a lot. Besides, that cat already has a home. He must live somewhere around here."

Jade ignored me. She started rubbing her chin against the cat's fur, saying, "Aah, you my sisser, kay?"

"Your sister? Oh, Jade, please don't do this to me."

The words "Mother" and "Guilt" were so closely entwined that I sometimes wondered what it would be like to go a whole week without denying Jade anything she wanted. But I drew some consolation in knowing that, at our old house which we shared with Jennifer, at least Jade had some pets: the field mice that invaded our humble abode.

Situated across from the Montreal West train station, the upper duplex we lived in was an old building in constant need of repair. The building trembled when a train went by—it sounded like it was tearing through our hallway. The landlord, his wife, and their two school-aged children lived below us. Our landlord was kind and extremely hardworking. We would often see him effecting repairs on the building, and he promptly obliged whenever we had any problems.

One fall morning, while I was preparing a snack of cheese and crackers, something scampered by. I stopped dead in my tracks, unsure whether I was imagining it, or if this house really did have other occupants. I saw it again. This time I freaked! Jade was in the living room watching *Sesame Street* when I swept her off the floor and held her tightly, to protect her from the horrible creature. I contemplated calling 9-1-1, but instead ran downstairs to find the landlord. He wasn't home.

I stood outside with Jade still in my arms, then spotted the landlord up on the scaffolding doing mortar work on the east brick wall. I called up to him, "There's a mouse in my house!" I couldn't believe his calmness as he simply replied, "Oh, that's typical at this time of year."

"Well?" I asked.

"I'll bring you some traps a little later."

The traps were set at nighttime. Jennifer was assigned the responsibility of disposals. She worked as an assistant bookkeeper at a funeral parlour, after all, so I hardly thought that a few dead mice would make her squeamish. We'd no sooner go to bed when we'd hear *snap, snap*. It seemed such a cruel thing to do, but what were our choices? Night after night, the same ritual. I'd hear the snap, call out, "Jennifer!" and she'd stomp down the hallway with a couple of expletives tripping off her tongue.

Eventually she muttered, "I'll take care of it in the morning." Not long after that, she said, "Forget it. What's the point? We no sooner get rid of a few, when a few more come in through the cracks and crevices of this building. Either that, or the horny little things are procreating."

Well, *I* wasn't about to assume the role of executioner, so man and mouse learned to live together as best we could. Sometimes, in the early morning, I'd hear the pitter patter of Jade's footsteps and then her sweetest, gentlest voice. "Oh, hi mousy."

When winter came, we still had some of our resident rodents. And why would they leave when they had it so good here? A nice warm house with plenty of food to eat. While Jennifer and I were very diligent about not leaving any food around, whenever I'd swept the floors, I'd find pieces of Jade's arrowroot biscuits hidden under the furniture in just about every room.

Sometimes we'd manage to corner the odd critter, leaving it no choice but to scuttle into the paper grocery bag, strategically set for this purpose. Then I'd ask Andrew to kindly escort it to the warm shelter of the train station. "We can't let it freeze to death," was my explanation. Somehow, I think Jade's fondness and respect for all living creatures had rubbed off on me.

Despite some of these problems, and despite the fact that the toilet was in one room and the rest of the bathroom in another, we loved this place since it had character, spacious rooms, high ceilings, and shiny hardwood floors in almost every room. So what that the kitchen was on a slant; Jade didn't mind this at all. She would sit on the highest grade of the linoleum floor, laughing wildly as her cars and trucks accelerated down the "ramp."

We were very happy living there, but it's a wonder we weren't evicted. I remember the day I bought a cheap, second-hand washing machine. I was as excited as a little kid with a brand new toy. No more doing laundry by hand, and no more wasting time at the laundromat. I plugged in the machine, and inserted the rubber hose into the drain pipe, not noticing that the lower part of the hose had a gaping crack in it. The first load of laundry was started.

We prepared supper, and as we were about to sit down to eat, there was a loud banging on our floor coming from the house below. Then the landlord charged upstairs and banged on the door. "Water is pouring through our kitchen ceiling!" he shouted.

I ran into the bathroom to discover a flood of sudsy water. Jennifer dashed downstairs to help clean up, while I grabbed every piece of linen I could get my hands on. A simple mopping wouldn't suffice in this situation. Jade stood in the bathroom doorway, shaking her head, not knowing what to make of all this mess. "Uh oh," she said. "Uh oh, Mommy, uh oh."

"Well don't just stand there, Jade, go find some other stuff to throw on the floor!" Jade then scurried off to her room to empty her dresser drawers.

When Jennifer returned, she said, "Gail, you should have seen it; it was awful, just awful! The whole family was sitting down to dinner when suddenly gobs of soap suds came plopping onto their plates. Water was seeping through the seams of the acoustic ceiling tiles; it was raining in their kitchen!"

Luckily, Andrew fixed the problem, and it never happened again.

At the first parent-teacher meeting, there were seven other mothers in the classroom who, like myself, were very eager to learn about their child's curriculum.

We were informed by the teacher, Janine, that the kids really loved each other and constantly kissed and hugged. "They are learning the 'Good Morning' song; they spend a lot of time learning how to recognize one another's names on cue cards; they hold brief discussions; they do arts and crafts, play games, and eventually they will be learning part of the alphabet and counting numbers up to five."

Each mother had her turn asking questions, all of which were satisfactorily answered. Everyone seemed to be satisfied with the curriculum—everyone except me. While making a comment to the teacher, I suddenly felt many disapproving stares. I had said to the teacher, "I hope that you will try to discourage the kids from eliciting so much constant affection." I went on, "As a mother, I am finding it increasingly difficult and frustrating to teach Jade to whom she can and cannot freely give her affection. It's not appropriate behaviour, especially when one's child goes up to a total stranger in a supermarket, giving him or her a big hug." I was about to say something else, when I was interrupted.

One offended mother said, "Our children are very loving children. Why would you want to change that?"

Another parent interjected, "You should accept your daughter as she is."

In an impatient, yet polite tone of voice, I argued, "If my child didn't approach a stranger, readily offering a hug, I certainly wouldn't consider her to be unloving. Outside of school, Jade has several friends. They don't run up to her, smothering her with kisses all the time, and I don't consider those kids to be unloving either. They're just acting in a normal, appropriate way."

Now I was getting even more impatient with this discussion. "Moreover, I do accept my child; however, what I do not accept is ignorance. If my child can learn to tug continuously on her ear and make weird sounds, a skill she recently learned, then she can learn to comply with adaptive behaviours as well."

I had further comments to make but decided to keep my mouth shut. When the meeting was over I stayed behind in the classroom to have a few private words with the teacher.

"Janine, when I had registered Jade for school, I was informed that the children placed in your class were of approximately the same level. It seems to me that if you are not yet teaching number counting and the alphabet, then Jade shouldn't be in your group, but rather in a more advanced class. Jade already knows the complete alphabet; she knows how to write most of the letters; she counts up to fifteen, and she is capable of sight-reading up to twenty practical words."

Janine replied, "It would be helpful, then, if you would provide me with a list of all the words Jade has learned, and I shall do my best to provide some extra time with Jade to help reinforce those reading skills."

My next question was, "Exactly where does Jade fit in with your class as far as language skills are concerned?"

"As far as language skills are concerned, Jade is the most verbal student in the class."

"So other than yourself and your assistant, Jade has nobody to model from, right?"

"Jade is doing just fine. She is happy in her class, participates in every activity, and maybe you're just expecting too much from her."

On the bus returning home, I couldn't stop thinking about the teacher's last remark—that I'm expecting too much from Jade. As I sat there deep in thought, I felt compelled to re-evaluate. I wasn't a pushy mother, the kind of mother I vowed I would never become, was I? I wasn't sure anymore. I kept thinking about it and decided that handicaps aside, Jade indeed was a bright child who, given the opportunity, was willing and eager to learn anything new. I was now so annoyed with myself, thinking of all the things I could have said—should have said—to the teacher, but didn't.

I couldn't sleep most of that night. I was too wired and worried about Jade. I wasn't satisfied with the education she was receiving or with the school's environment. I wanted to change the situation but didn't know how. I tossed and turned, trying to think of a better plan for Jade but couldn't come up with anything.

Somehow, I felt that Jade and I were losing some of the closeness we had always shared. There just wasn't enough time in a day, but since Jade spent so much time at school and so much time commuting, it was understandable that she'd be too tired to do anything afterward.

If we weren't spending our Saturdays with Andrew, Jade and I usually went to the park. But it just wasn't the same. Jade saw some of the familiar faces from summer day camp, but those children had since formed many of their own friendships at the neighbourhood school. They had moved together in the same direction, from nursery school to day camp to kindergarten, and Jade was now only a summertime friend, if in fact they still wanted her around next summer.

I then decided that Jade should also have school friends with whom she could play with outside of the school's environment. I contacted the mother of one of Jade's classmates and invited her daughter, Marianne, for an afternoon visit.

Jade was delighted at the prospect of having one of her classmates over to play. When Marianne arrived, she totally ignored Jade and instead dashed around the house for no apparent reason. She laughed and screamed, then tried to spoon the two fish out of the fish bowl. Jade was becoming annoyed and somewhat frustrated. "No Mayanne, toppit! No hutt *Fishy* and *Boot!* You *no* my fend!" she shouted.

I took out some of Jade's favourite board games and tried to entice both girls into playing something quiet, but no such luck. Marianne was now in the bathroom, flushing and flushing the toilet. "No, Mayanne," Jade continued, in a very stern voice.

Jade was angry, stormed into her bedroom, and slammed the door behind her, yelling, "Lee me lone! No bugging me, you toopid oss!"

I know it wasn't funny, but I had to laugh anyway. It was the first time I ever heard Jade call someone a stupid ass.

When I stopped laughing, I had to hurry off to see what

Marianne was up to next. Jade, I thought, I need your help. Don't abandon me now. Marianne's mother is not due back for another two hours.

Jade stayed alone in her room until Marianne left, and I couldn't blame her. I was so exhausted that I promised myself: never, ever again!

I received a telephone call from Evelyn (Evy) Lusthaus. She was the mother of Hannah, the little girl who was integrated into regular day care, the same little girl who had opened the door to Jade regarding day care. Evy was very interested in meeting with other parents of intellectually challenged children, in order to share some of our experiences. With so much in common, we spoke for about an hour. I gladly accepted the invitation to meet with her and the other parents.

In all, we were six mothers: Evy, Joan (Jade's former foster mother), Agnes Wee, Rissa Mechaly, Madeleine Engel, and me. We each took turns speaking about our children's school experiences. We also talked about our frustrations and hopes about our children's education. Like me, everyone was dissatisfied with the education their children were currently receiving. Though Hannah attended regular kindergarten, no special assistance was provided. All the other children were being educated in segregated special schools.

We agreed to meet regularly as an aid and support to one another—our main goal being the integration of our children into the regular neighbourhood schools.

This mutual goal, however, was going to require a lot of consistent teamwork. It meant gathering information about what was available for our children in the regional school boards and trying to get an understanding of the school system and the special services offered. It meant meeting with school board officials, special education teachers, and various consultants, and it would involve attending any conferences that might be scheduled concerning school integration. We all had a common interest, and we all had great hopes for what we could accomplish by working together as a team.

In one of our many meetings with school board officials, we learned that most school principals and staff did not have any knowledge or understanding of Down syndrome and other forms of mental retardation, and this resulted in a negative outlook on the subject of integration. Hence, our group's next step was to relay as much information as possible concerning children with mental handicaps.

We received some encouraging information at an integration seminar, sponsored by the Quebec Institute on Mental Retardation. Their philosophies included:

> Whatever a child's ability or disability, he or she is to be educated. Not special education, but education. Education is to foster growth, and we believe that all kids can grow. All children need to belong, be accepted, affirm each other, and experience success.

> Segregation does not work. Children learn more from each other than from themselves. We all need models. The comment, "a six-to-one ratio in education is good education," is not right. That is instruction, not education. Integration enhances dignity and produces growth. It is a double learning experience. Exceptional pupils should enjoy the benefits of schooling with their brothers and sisters in their own neighbourhood school.

This was like music to our ears—our sentiments exactly. And after listening to success stories, how could we settle for less? We heard stories about schools that had integrated a child with challenging needs. We heard about how each of these schools later reported that they had since become a better school. Children touched children whom they normally wouldn't have had contact with. These kids would grow up with values and attitudes they wouldn't have necessarily acquired otherwise.

After attending a couple of these conferences, Evy, whom we jokingly called the brain of our group, compiled the information and ideas that we each submitted to her, then completed a very detailed and thoroughly researched proposal regarding school integration. We deliberated carefully, and when all the points had been agreed upon, we presented the proposal to our school board.

Outlined in our proposal were the exact steps that could be taken in order that children with mental retardation could receive their education in an age-appropriate regular class in a neighbourhood school, with specialized support services made available to them, and to the regular class teacher. We stated our beliefs:

- That both children with retardation and children who are normal benefit from being educated together in a rich, accepting cooperative environment;
- That the development of children with retardation is enhanced when they have consistent, positive interactions with normal children, and that the development of normal children is enhanced when they have consistent, positive interaction with children who have special needs;
- That the key to success for the integration of children with special needs is the willingness and commitment of those involved. This includes school principal, classroom teacher, support personnel, parents and children, and the creative use of volunteers, among others;
- That the educational programs for children with retardation need to be planned, structured, and evaluated in careful, systematic ways;
- That the regular teachers must be supported in getting the help they need in order to make integration a success;
- That parents have the right and responsibility to be involved in their children's educational programs.

Certain school board officials were in total agreement with the concept of our integration proposal, but many more discussions were to be held amongst all levels of the school system. Our parents' group was subsequently elected to act as a

106

subcommittee, working in conjunction with the board on this project, which involved many more months of planning and organizing.

All the while, Jade remained at her segregated school.

CHAPTER ELEVEN

For Jade, a common cold often meant a trip to the pediatrician's office. She was terrified of doctors and their medical instruments; she cringed at absolutely anything that would be used during even the simplest of examinations. Actually, there was no such thing as a simple examination. Even the scale posed a threat to Jade. Her weight, more often than not, had to be "guesstimated."

No matter how many attempts had been made to reassure Jade of her safety, her screams were blood-curdling. She refused to let the doctor get close to her, let alone touch her, and with all of her strength, she kicked and screamed. Any attempts to restrain her frightened her that much more, to the point that her whole body would shake. It was such an overwhelming experience that I trembled almost as much as Jade. Seeing her in such distress, feeling her feelings of helplessness, I hurt so much that I just couldn't find the courage to hold back my own tears.

One November night, I was awakened by a strange noise, an unfamiliar sound, like a barking seal. I sat up in bed wondering if I had been dreaming. The barking started again. I got up, trying to detect where the noise was coming from. I went into Jade's room. She was sitting up in her bed, gasping for breath. Her face was puffy, and there was blueness about her mouth and fingernails. I felt her forehead. She was burning with fever, her hair soaking with sweat.

I rushed to the bathroom to get a cool, damp cloth and a glass of water. After spending a few minutes with her, trying to figure out what was wrong, I telephoned the hospital's emergency room and described what was happening.

We arrived at the hospital around midnight. Because

Jade's name was a permanent entry on the hospital's priority list, our waiting time was minimal.

When the battle between Jade and the doctor was over, I was informed that Jade had come down with a dangerous form of croup, a viral infection of the voice box. The treatment included hospitalization and intensive antibiotic therapy.

Due to Jade's heart disorder, the doctors decided that she should be kept under close observation in the intensive care unit. Jade and I were met on that ward by one of Cardiology's resident doctors, Dr. Bertrand. The doctor said, "Jade has already been under so much stress that I am not going to re-examine her without her consent. I was informed by the emergency doctor what to expect from Jade, and I don't want to upset her—it'll only make matters worse."

I spent the night at Jade's bedside, watching as her colour returned to a healthy shade of pink, thanks to the oxygen tent. I must have fallen asleep in the chair when I heard the voice of a little kid saying, "Shh, shh, Mommy seepin." I looked up and saw a nurse standing by Jade's bed. Then the screaming started. Jade crawled back into the oxygen tent and tried to hide behind a pillow.

The nurse attempted to persuade Jade to cooperate. "Please, Jade," she said, "I just want to take your temperature. It won't hurt a bit."

"No temchur," Jade pleaded. "Go way!"

My assistance was required again. God, how I hated feeling like the enemy! I did my best to console Jade, all the while holding her arms and legs in place so she couldn't fight off the nurse.

While Jade was napping that afternoon, I went home to shower and change. When I returned to the hospital, Jade was again trying to hide in the oxygen tent, screaming, "No touchin me! Lee me lone!" There were three young interns trying to examine her.

Instinctively, I acted in Jade's defence. "Why is she getting more examinations?" I demanded to know. "Where is Dr. Bertrand, Jade's doctor?"

I was then told that these checkups were merely routine, a teaching tool for interns.

"Listen," I said, "I know you need the hands-on experience, but *not* with my child. Where is Dr. Bertrand? I want to make sure that nobody needlessly upsets Jade."

The interns obliged and told me that they would inform the doctor of my wishes.

Obviously proud of me, Jade started to cheer. "Yay, Mommy!" With her arms outstretched, she asked for a hug. I was then rewarded with about ten big kisses on the cheek. "Good ger, Mommy," she praised me. "You good ger."

Three days later, she was well enough to return home.

Andrew was very concerned and sympathetic to the rough time Jade had been through. In view of all the damp, cold weather we'd been having, he generously offered to help pay our expenses so we could join him on a trip to Florida, where he had a place to stay.

So that Jade wouldn't get overly tired, we brought her stroller everywhere with us—just in case. We had an unforgettable vacation showing Jade some of the main attractions, such as the Weeki Wachi Mermaid show, horse and bird shows, and Dwarf Village, an amusement park for young children.

We spent a couple of hours wandering around a tropical rain forest, and surprisingly, Jade never seemed to tire. She loved the freedom and the wondrous discoveries of nature. I was amused to observe Jade talking to a parrot perched on a tree branch. She was trying to get it to repeat her words. "Fish," she'd say, but the bird wouldn't respond.

Next, we went on a picnic—Jade's favourite dining experience—at Pine Island Beach. For about five minutes, Jade actually sat down to eat. She then grabbed a celery stick and wandered off to meet new people.

Later, Jade went into the water to practice her swimming.

She lay in the shallow water and, using her arms, she'd pull her body forward, yelling, "Wook Andu! Wook Gayo! I wimmin! Watchin me! Watchin me!" Andrew and I couldn't take our eyes off her for a minute—we weren't allowed to.

Among other things, Jade had the opportunity to drive a Jade-sized automobile. She tried out several vehicles, then spotted something she thought to be more fun. She rolled around on a huge, tented air cushion that was covered with thousands of plastic Ping Pong balls. It was a riot to watch her! Her whole body was covered with green Ping Pong balls, then out popped her head. She held up one of the balls, looked at Andrew and me, saying, "Pay baw, an-one?"

"Yes, Jade," I laughed. "We'd love to play ball with you, but we're not allowed to join you in there, because we're too big."

Trying to sound sincere, Jade said in a sweet, sympathetic voice, "Aah, too bad. Mayme nex time." She started to laugh and immersed herself into the mass of Ping Pong balls, squealing with delight.

Smiling at me, Andrew sarcastically remarked, "What a phony, that kid of yours!"

The next attraction was Busch Gardens' petting zoo. We no sooner got past the entrance gate when Jade was about ten yards ahead of us. The goats and sheep took one quick glance at Jade and her ice-cream cone, then came running toward her. "No no!" she screamed. "Go way! You bad boys! Go way!"

This was all happening within thirty fast seconds, and by the time Andrew and I caught up to Jade, the ice cream was on the ground, the animals were ravenously gulping it down, and with tears coursing down her cheeks, Jade cried, "Wanna go home now, Mommy." Of course, we stayed a while longer but that was only possible because Andrew agreed to Jade's request that she sit atop his shoulders.

One evening, while Jade and Andrew were watching television, Jade noticed a fly buzzing around the room. Andrew told her where the fly swatter was, but instead Jade went into the kitchen and got a package of crackers. She returned, offered some to Andrew, then asked the whereabouts of the fly. A few minutes later the fly reappeared, and Jade tried to get a closer look at it. She snapped off a small piece of cracker and offered it to the fly.

Our next and final visit was to Walt Disney's Magic Kingdom, where we met many wonderful characters. Jade didn't think they were so wonderful, though. "Too big an cawey," she'd say as she pulled away when I tried to bring her up close to meet them. That wasn't going to stop me, though. After all, how often does one get the chance to meet Goofy, Donald Duck, and the Three Bears in person? Jade was content as long as she was at a safe distance from these so-called scary characters.

She also found the first rides we went on to be "too dock an cawey," and she'd bury her head in my lap. But when we took the boat ride through the tunnel called, "It's a Small World (After All)", Jade was impressed by the display of colourful, dancing dolls, each representing a country of the world. She especially enjoyed the happy music and, after we came out of the tunnel, continued to sing, "Maw woo atta awe, maw woo atta awe . . ." At Jade's request, we took this ride for a second, then a third time.

We went on the "Jungle Cruise," which turned out to be Jade's favourite. "One moe time," she insisted as we exited the ride, "Juss one moe time".

As we headed toward the exit of Disney World, we heard an announcement over the loud speaker: "It's Donald Duck's fiftieth birthday today, and you are all invited to celebrate his birthday."

We decided to stay a while longer; we couldn't very well let Jade miss out on this. There was a grand parade and Jade loved anything that attracted crowds of people, and the music thrilled her so. As the entire Disney clan paraded down the streets, singing "Happy Birthday to Donald Duck," Jade excitedly joined in. Alice in Wonderland skipped over to greet this ecstatic kid. She gave Jade a hug, then handed her a red balloon. Jade was laughing, applauding, and screaming. "Oh, Yay! Donna Duck's boo-day! Hooway!"

Christmas was coming soon, another greatly anticipated holiday to enjoy with my precious daughter. While Andrew was in the process of building a wooden dump truck for Jade, I was creating a photo album for her. It included all of the photographs of our Florida vacation, each picture having a funny little caption that best described the moment.

About a week before Christmas, we started to decorate the house. Jade drew many pictures of Santa, reindeer, and Christmas trees, and taped each picture onto the lower part of the walls of every room. The Christmas records played over and over again with Jade happily singing along.

Eager to help with gift-wrapping, Jade wanted to know what gift was for whom, then assured me: "Gamma wuv diss. David wuv diss. An I wuv kissmas!"

This was also the year when the Cabbage Patch Kid was all the rage. Tipped off about new shipments to arrive, people were lined up for blocks, shivering in the frigid winter cold, just waiting for the stores to open their doors. While this toy of the year ranked high on Jade's wish list, I wasn't about to camp out overnight to make it happen. When Jade opened one of her gift boxes on Christmas morning, she trembled with excitement. I don't know how Jim and Joan had managed it, but Jade received her very own Cabbage Patch doll.

Jade was happy to go to mass to celebrate Jesus' birthday. We then went with Andrew to my parents' house for the traditional turkey dinner. Jade spent most of the afternoon sorting through the many gifts under the large, beautifully decorated spruce tree in the living room. She carefully sifted through each pile of gifts, seeking those labels that had her name on them. With a look of disappointment on her face, Jade came to see me in the kitchen: "No pesents Jade, Mommy."

"Are you sure, Jade?" I asked. "Did you look really carefully?"

She shrugged her shoulders, then confirmed, "No pesents Jade. Aah well."

Then the doorbell rang. Finally. The cameras were ready. As Jade opened the door, we heard a scream. "Santa Cause! Santa Cause!" As she was motioning this terrific person to come inside the house, she called out to Poppa, "Santa Cause here, Poppa! Fasser, fasser, comin see!" That was the moment we were all anticipating—the surprised, happy look on Jade's face.

Santa pulled the gifts out of his big red bag and handed them to each of the kids. Jade thanked him a thousand times, then just stood there by his side, her eyes wide open. She hadn't even attempted to unwrap the gifts. Santa's very presence was enough for her.

CHAPTER TWELVE

Bearing in mind Jade's upcoming cardiology appointment, I tried to determine a way to help her overcome her fear of doctors. For me, the stress started to build up days ahead of the appointment, and although Jade and I had often played doctor, the plastic, colourful instruments did not closely enough resemble the actual medical instruments.

As a matter of fact, even a simple haircut posed a threat to Jade. I remember the day I nicked her eyebrow while trying to trim her bangs, as she forcefully pushed my hand away. I felt so awful about it and still feel guilty to this day. From then on, I would trim Jade's hair while she was sleeping and she would wake up with these incredibly crooked bangs that I would later ask my sister to fix during a subsequent nap.

Although I hadn't any urgent medical requirement of my own, I nonetheless set up a couple of appointments where the roles would be reversed. Jade was going to be the onlooker.

I explained to the dentist beforehand my intentions. Sitting on a stool alongside the dentist chair, Jade attentively watched my calm reactions as the dentist cleaned and checked my teeth. "See, Jade, it didn't hurt at all," I said. Jade started giggling, then said apprehensively, "No me!"

Of course, anything more than a basic checkup, and this whole plan would have backfired. The saying, "The apple doesn't fall far from the tree," couldn't be more true in this case. When I was a child, a dentist became so nervous and frustrated with all my carrying on that he actually slapped me across the face. My mother promptly found a new dentist. And I wasn't any more cooperative when it came to vaccinations.

There were two sets of eyes staring into my mouth. One person was trying to clean my teeth while the other was trying to count them. Afterward, the dentist persuaded Jade to open her mouth, and she agreed—for about half a second. Jade left the office with a brand new toothbrush, a small tube of toothpaste, and a big smile. My plan is working, I thought. No tears—for either of us.

The next appointment, Jade accompanied me to the dermatologist's office, where I had a minor biopsy performed on my foot. "See, Jade, it doesn't hurt a bit," I said, as I jerked at the sight of the needle, trying not to scream.

"Dottor make betta, eh, Mommy?"

"Oh yes, Jade, I feel much better now."

The cardiology appointment proved to be a much more pleasant visit this time around. Jade was slightly more trusting of the medical staff. She even managed to crack a smile when the examination was completed.

"There has been no change," Dr. Gibbons stated. "As you know, the condition of Jade's heart is not going to improve; however, there are no signs of further deterioration, which of course is good. No heart medication is necessary and won't be required until such time as her heart condition worsens, and there is no way of telling when that might be. Jade seems to be doing very well, and my advice to you is to keep doing whatever it is you're doing. Jade can participate in all activities, providing she doesn't strain herself and get overtired."

Jade seemed quite content to return to school after the holidays, but there hadn't been any noticeable progress in her language, or in her gross and fine motor skills. I had inquired at the school once before about language therapy but learned that Jade was not able to get such therapy. There was only one speech therapist and some two hundred students. "There are many other students who are in greater need," I was informed, "and it is only these priority

116

students who are able to receive such a service."

Why, I wondered, was Jade going to a *special* school then?

I arranged for a couple of all-day visits with the school in order to observe Jade and what she was learning. I wanted to obtain a clear picture of the whole school day, starting with the ride to school in the morning.

Jade was so proud to have me seated next to her on the school bus. An older child, about ten or eleven years of age, started yelling out a couple of words that I couldn't understand. She continued chanting these two words all the way to school, with Jade repeating them.

A few children were excitedly awaiting the driver's next stop. There were a couple of four- or five-year-olds who sat quietly, seemingly unaware of what was going on around them, and at the rear of the bus, a couple of teenagers were in a heated argument over something.

When we arrived at school, Jade anxiously escorted me to her classroom. She introduced me to her classmates, then headed to her chair. When all the children were seated, the teachers began to sing a song. A few of the kids were mumbling along, while Jade, with a big grin, kept turning her head to the back of the class to make sure I was still there.

I accompanied Jade to her twenty-minute physiotherapy program, which I learned was nothing more than the simple exercises we do at home each day. I guess it was the term, physiotherapy, that made me think it required a highly qualified professional to teach these exercises.

Back in the classroom, it was mainly free-play, and there was very little in the way of instruction.

On the next visit to Jade's school, I not only observed Jade throughout the day, but I also paid closer attention to the environment. It really was an institution, I thought. My heart went out to Jade as well as to all the other children, for they had no one to model from but themselves. These children were leading such a nonstimulating life, I thought. How could they function later on in the real world? But Jade was my main concern.

At the next school meeting, I brought it to the teacher's attention that I felt it was important to provide more instruction in Jade's curriculum. I advised her of my plans and efforts to integrate Jade into a regular school the following year, and I added that Jade needed better preparation.

The teacher was shocked. "Integrate! How could you do that to her? Jade is doing just fine here, and she would only regress if you stick her in a large classroom with normal children."

I told her about the parents' group I had been meeting with, the conferences I had attended, and the research our group had carried out. But it was clear that she was reluctant even to try to understand my viewpoint, as she continued to shake her head negatively.

Just then, the school's social worker walked into the classroom to sit in on the meeting. The teacher, still on the defensive, said, "Jade will be ridiculed and rejected if she is integrated into a regular class. The other children will make fun of her, and she will probably end up in a corner somewhere crying."

At this point, I was near tears. The social worker was quick to catch on to our conversation and added, "What, integrate Jade! Oh, don't tell me you're thinking of putting Jade in a regular school. Integration *never* works. The handicapped child *always* suffers. In a regular school, Jade would be deprived of the special services that she desperately needs in order to help her learn."

I argued, "How could you say that? Exactly what so-called special services is Jade receiving here? As far as I understand, Jade is the most verbal pupil in her class, with no one to model from. But is she receiving language stimulation through the services of a speech therapist? No, she isn't."

I then added, "Jade has some gross motor problems and, yes, she is receiving physiotherapy. Some of it, though—basic exercises, which take about an hour each week—could easily be done at home. And, in fact, they are."

The social worker argued back, "But there are other

things, such as the expertise of a special education teacher. There's also a very small student-teacher ratio here, which you won't find in a regular school."

"Fine," I said, "a good ratio and special education—then why haven't I noticed any progress in Jade's development?"

The teacher interjected, "If Jade were my child, I would definitely keep her in this school. She is happy here with other children who are just like her."

Now I was ready to explode. "First of all," I said, "Jade is not your child and, no, she is not just like all the other children. Each individual child is unique, in case you hadn't noticed. You make me sound like a cruel, uncaring mother, and I don't appreciate it. I would never, ever, make changes in Jade's life that I thought would cause her to regress. I know my child better than anyone else does, and I obviously have higher expectations of her than you do. Furthermore, you make 'normal' children sound like horrible monsters, just waiting for the opportunity to pounce on my child."

I couldn't believe my assertiveness—I never knew I had it in me. Whereas once I was passive, following any direction in which someone would lead or drag me, I was now an advocate, an activist, a true fighter—fighting for what I believed in. And I have to say it was a really good feeling, an empowering feeling.

In a calmer voice, I tried to explain once again the philosophy and benefits of integration, but I could see I was still getting nowhere.

I didn't sleep the entire night, just tossed and turned and worried. I felt trapped. Jade's future. It was such an important decision to make. On the one hand, I had the same feelings and goals as the parents in our support group. There was mutual encouragement and a school board decision soon to be made. On the other hand, I was being painted a heartbreaking picture of a dejected little girl who was going to regress, secluding herself into an unhappy corner of the world.

I started to question my role as a mother. Was I being objective? Was I being over-demanding? Was I trying to satisfy my needs, or Jade's needs, or both?

In April, Jade was sent home from school with a fair-sized bruise on her head as well as a fractured collarbone. My neighbour, who was to baby-sit that day, met her at the bus. The driver said that Jade was crying on the bus and that a teacher had mentioned to him that she had been crying that afternoon. The baby-sitter paid immediate attention to Jade and, within five minutes, recognized the severity of the bump on Jade's head and her bruised, swollen shoulder. Jade was immediately transported to a medical clinic, which in turn advised that she be taken to the hospital for x-rays.

When I met up with them at the hospital, Jade cried, "Tony pushing me foor, faw down."

"Oh, poor Jade," I sympathized. "Where were you when Tony pushed you?"

"Toyette," she cried, "Tony pushing me toyette. Tony a bad boy."

From this message, I presumed that Jade was pushed off the side of the toilet onto her right side, also lacerating the skin above her eye, possibly on the paper holder.

Because the school hadn't contacted the baby-sitter or me, I asked the physician if it was usual for a child to break a collarbone and feel no pain. I was told that it was highly unlikely unless the child was in shock, but in all probability, the signs of shock would have been indicated.

Because there was dried blood on Jade's forehead when she arrived home from school, it was obvious that it had to have bled earlier that day. I read the teacher's note that was in Jade's lunch box:

> Just before going home, we saw the little bruise on Jade's head (over the eye). We think it happened in the bathroom, but she was not crying when she fell there. Hope she forgets it quickly.

But with a shoulder brace and the constant assistance required, neither Jade nor I forgot it too quickly.

120

Jade was home from school for almost a month and I started to work for another company in the evenings, while my downstairs neighbour stayed with Jade. Jade came to love the new routine of having me home with her all day, and having the time to play with the old board games that had been forgotten for a while. She thrived on routine, making certain that I adhered to it. At about eight o'clock every morning, Jade came to wake me. She'd crawl into my bed, massage my back a while, then give me a kiss on the cheek, saying, "Good monning, Mommy, time get up, I hugwee."

While I showered and dressed, Jade would wait patiently at the kitchen table. Each morning, without fail, she was in a cheerful, humorous mood. When breakfast was finished she'd always remember to ask for her vitamins.

I was so proud that Jade was learning to be quite self-sufficient. Everything she needed in the bathroom was set at a reachable level, and she took care of her own personal hygiene as any child her age would. She liked to choose her clothing each day and dressed herself without assistance—although these days, she needed some assistance due to the shoulder brace.

We went out for a walk each morning, and upon our return, Jade would watch *Sesame Street*, one of her favourite television programs. It was a program that reinforced a lot of what I was teaching her. Whenever we were at the supermarket, Jade eagerly pointed out any familiar words and numbers on the advertising signs.

Each afternoon, Jade and I would spend a couple of hours sitting at her desk, fitting puzzles, colouring, reading, and playing card games. For Jade, there never seemed to be a boring moment. If I was preoccupied with other things, she always found something to do on her own. When playing with her toys, Jade used her imagination to the fullest, acting out teacher, doctor, football coach, camp counsellor, or mommy.

Music was also a large and interesting part of her life. She often played records and danced around with her dolls. She loved music so much, in fact, that each evening she would choose a tape for her tape recorder, which was placed on the bathroom floor, so she could sing along while bathing.

Music was also the only issue that got Jade and me into a battle of wills. I mean, there's only so much *Skinnamarink* one could listen to before going out in public and getting caught singing the same song you're trying to shake off. When the voices of Sharon, Lois and Bram, or Raffi weren't filling the house, I might be lucky enough to play some of my own music. I'd be cleaning the house with either hard rock or reggae blasting away, when suddenly the music switched to the ever-entertaining "Turkey in the Straw," with Jade lip-synching into a soup ladle-*cum*-microphone. While Jade had her own portable record player, my stereo was her hi-fi of choice, since it had speakers. Stubborn as *I* could be, Jade nonetheless won out every time.

Bedtime was always special—for both of us. Most nights, anticipating story time, Jade was delighted to go to bed. She usually requested "pesho" stories—my own stories, in which she was the main character: the heroine who managed to locate the missing bread at the grocery store, or the champion who discovered the hidden treasure in the sandbox. Without exception, every story had to begin with: "Once upon a time, there was a little girl named Jade . . ." She especially enjoyed these anecdotes because they covered the day's events in great exaggeration, and if I left anything out, she was quick to add her own version.

We then prayed, starting with the "Lord's Prayer," then offering our own personal prayer. Jade no sooner finished God-blessing the whole world when she'd peacefully fall asleep.

I'd check in on her at least three times a night, each time thanking God for such a wonderful, precious gift. Upon retiring to my own bed, I'd reminisce, for each day spent with Jade was usually a treasury of fond memories. I thought mostly of the constant amusement that only Jade could provide. I'd chuckle over something she had said that day, or what she had done that morning, or the message she had relayed over the telephone.

I thought about an incident that happened a while ago: One day I was too sick to get out of bed. When Jade came into my room that morning, I tried to get up, but everything went pitch black. I had a terrible flu and was too weak to even get to the phone to call for a baby-sitter, or anyone who might be able to help out. I slept for hours at a time. At each waking interval, and after a quick dash to the bathroom, I was greeted by a caring, young nurse who tried everything to make me better. If memory serves, at one time she brought me a cup of water, then a slice of buttered bread, then her bottle of vitamins, then a bowl of applesauce.

Each time she'd say, "Get betta, Mommy, kay? Get betta. I watchin TV now." Then I'd receive a kiss on the forehead. "See ya wader, Mommy."

By six o'clock that evening I was finally able to get out of bed. My God! I realized that Jade had been on her own all day. I went into the living room where all of Jade's board games had been set up. The television was on, and a Sharon, Lois and Bram tape filled the room, drowning out the evening news.

The bathroom had been disinfected with Vaseline petroleum jelly. Two dolls, with Halloween makeup applied to their faces, were seated on the toilet.

I went into the kitchen and noted that Jade, fortunately, hadn't starved that day. Better still, from the traces of food I saw, she had eaten well indeed: alfalfa sprouts, muffins, cheese, tomato juice, and butter—lots of butter.

I then went into Jade's bedroom and saw her sitting quietly, contentedly, in front of the full-length mirror. The room was fairly dark and she hadn't thought about turning on the lights. She was wearing one of the many costumes from her dress-up box. I just stood there, watching this innocent, self-sufficient creature, waiting for her to notice me. She spotted me in the mirror, then turned to me, exclaiming, "Oh Mommy, you up! You up! I so happy! You betta now?"

Before giving me a chance to answer, Jade pointed to her painted face, "Wookit, I a funny cown!"

"You certainly are a funny clown, Jade. I love you. You were such a good girl today. So responsible! You did everything all by yourself, and I'm so proud of you!"

She beamed. "Yeah, I a big girl."

"My stomach is still a little upset," I explained, "but maybe I'll feel better if I eat some soup. Can you help me make it?"

"Yeah, Mommy, you sick," she answered, "I make it."

When we sat down to eat, I took the package of bread, and as I reached for the butter dish, Jade said, "No, Mommy, did it weddy. I butta it weddy."

In fact, the entire loaf of bread had been pre-buttered. Trying to put an appreciative smile on my face, I simply said, "Oh, Jade, you really were a busy girl today. Now we won't have to bother buttering our bread for a whole week."

"I big hepp eh, Mommy?"

"Yup, you sure are a big help."

By early May, I had no doubts whatsoever concerning my plans for Jade's education. My decision had been firmly, positively made. Jade would not be returning to the special school, whether or not she was accepted into the regular school. If, for whatever reasons, the school board did not accept the integration proposal, I fully intended to keep Jade at home. I'd teach her myself, I determined, but not without a fight first. I'd take my case to court if I had to. Jade had every right to be a part of her community, and that included her community school.

Later on that month, our parents' group was advised of the school board's decision. Jade and two other students with special needs were accepted at Elizabeth Ballantyne Elementary, our neighbourhood school—with the provision of support services, while the other children in our group were being accepted into their own local schools.

Another goal achieved! By the end of the month Jade had met her new kindergarten teacher, Miss Ingrid Klein, the special education teacher, Mrs. Linda Mahler, as well as the school's principal, Mrs. Elizabeth Kremmel.

As the five of us sat in the kindergarten classroom discussing Jade's skills, Jade was busy exploring. She drew pictures on the chalkboard, checked out the books and toys, then found her way to the playhouse. Jade was especially impressed with the playhouse, so much so that she didn't want to leave when the interview was over.

After meeting with the school's staff and feeling reassured of their acceptance and willingness to accommodate Jade, I became even more confident that this environment was going to provide a lot of positive learning.

As Jade and I walked home, we talked about her new school and her new teachers.

"I wike it," she said. "Morrow scoo, kay, Mommy?"

"No, Jade," I replied, "there's no school tomorrow. It's finished for the year, but you can go to day camp this summer, and then you can go to your new school when camp is finished."

"Oh yeah, camp? Oh hank you, Mommy, hank you."

Day camp to Jade was what summer was all about. Her mornings were spent with a group of children who sang songs, played games, and went on mini-excursions.

Each day as Jade bid her friends good-bye, she noticed that some of the kids were being met by their fathers. This bothered her for she knew that this was a person who was missing in her own life, and although she was happy to see me when I arrived at the campsite, she couldn't help but observe the children who were driven home by their dads. She said, "Wan daddy pick up fer wunch, kay, Mommy?"

I explained to her that not all children had fathers who lived with them, and we didn't have a choice in the matter. While I didn't want to brush aside the topic, I simply didn't know how to delve into the details of the marriage breakup. How could I ever expect her to understand? I had to look for the positive and hope that it would be satisfactory. "But we're a happy family, aren't we, Jade?" Jade wasn't buying it. She wanted a father just as the other kids had, and that was perfectly normal and perfectly understandable.

After lunch and a short nap, Jade would spend most of the afternoon at the park or at the large public swimming pool. She loved the water, and this year she was brave enough to jump off the side of the pool. "Catchin me," she screamed. "No ferget!" Then, holding onto my arms, she swam around, yelling to anyone in sight: "Wookit me, I wimmin!"

Other times, we'd go to the wading pool, where Jade would lay on the pool's cement floor and pull herself around until her legs and stomach were chafed. This didn't seem to bother her, though, because she was, after all, swimming.

She was usually well-accepted by other children she met, but still, there were kids who weren't so accepting, and those were the times that I sometimes wished I didn't have to be around. Yet it was a part of life. It hurt me to watch Jade when she'd approach a group of kids only to be ignored, or worse, asked why she talked like a baby and had funny eyes.

But for young children it was understandable, because they simply didn't know better. Sometimes, I tried to explain to them that God had made Jade a little differently, that Jade was special, that she took a little longer to learn things, but that she was also like other children. She liked to play, and she liked to make new friends. The children usually accepted this explanation. If only certain parents could have been as understanding.

My heart always went out to Jade when I'd see a mother whisk away her young child, simply because Jade came too close. It was as if some people thought that whatever Jade had might be contagious. And it was times like those that I just wanted to hold Jade in my arms, protecting her from society's cruel and cold ignorance.

Speaking of ignorance, I can't remember how many times other mothers asked me this question: "If you ever become pregnant again and you're offered an amniocentesis, and the result is Down syndrome, would you abort?" It was a question that required no contemplation to answer. I'd sigh, then throw the question right back at them. "You know this little child of yours that you personally gave birth to, this child who grew and kicked inside your body, this child you love with your whole heart and soul, this child you would lay down your life for—would *you* abort?"

Jim and Joan had moved and now lived in our neighbourhood, which gave Jade and Emmanuel ample opportunities to visit with each other. Emmanuel, now a stocky, athletic ten-year-old, continued to enjoy Jade's company. His speech wasn't very clear, and I often had trouble understanding him. Jade, however, had no problem; they communicated clearly and freely with one another. The laughter they shared was enough to make anyone laugh along.

The summertime, with all its warmth and freshness, did wonders for Jade. She had a terrific appetite, a good strong build, bright blue eyes, a healthy pink complexion, and soft blonde hair that now had golden highlights from the sun. To further enhance Jade's physical appearance, I always dressed her in the latest fashion in clothing, much of it in pretty pastel shades. "She's the picture of health," people would say to me—and that was the greatest compliment I could ever receive.

Aside from Jim and Joan, and people who had *had* to be informed of Jade's heart problem, nobody else knew. This privacy was for my own protection, I decided—a way to avoid the inevitable questions that go along with the mention of a heart condition. I worried that even the most well-intentioned people might possibly strike a sensitive nerve.

Since the end of day camp, school was all Jade could talk about. A week before school started, the two of us went to the shopping plaza to purchase some new school clothing. At a children's store, among all the clothing on the racks, Jade spotted a plaid jumper that really appealed to her.

"Buy diss fer me, kay, Mommy?"

We then chose a cream coloured blouse to go with the jumper, socks, leotards, underwear, and then a couple of outfits. As we stood at the cash to pay for the items, Jade smilingly looked up at the saleswoman and said, "New scoo cose. I happy. Go at scoo nex week."

Jade took the parcels from my hand. "My scoo cose, I'm carry dem." She then entered the adjacent shoe store and

127

instructed the sales clerk, "New shoes, pease. Bue." I wasn't even planning on her getting new shoes but, well, I had to.

Excited and nervous, Jade had trouble sleeping the night before school. While I was relaxing in the living room, I heard Jade talking to herself and to her dolls. "Scoo morrow. New teacher—Miss Kine." She chatted and giggled nervously for at least an hour before finally falling asleep.

I had trouble sleeping that night as well, for I had become just as excited and nervous as Jade. I felt great satisfaction that Jade had only a short walk to school each day, rather than having to spend so much time on a bus. I anticipated her making new friends who belonged to our neighbourhood, and I greatly anticipated the learning that would take place merely by Jade's being in a normal environment.

But I also worried. What if the staff at the segregated school proved to be correct in their prediction that Jade would regress? What if Jade was subjected to ridicule and rejection? What if Jade was miserable in her new surroundings? After tossing and turning for hours, I finally resolved to forget the "what ifs." Should the worst scenario become a reality, I'll deal with it then.

When I awoke the following morning, Jade was already dressed for school. I made her some breakfast, but she refused to eat. I didn't push the issue—it was the first day jitters, I presumed.

Jade returned to her bedroom to observe herself in the full-length mirror. With a big grin, she turned to me: "I wook nice, eh, Mommy?"

"Absolutely, Jade." I said. "You look beautiful. Such nice new clothes."

"New shoes, too," she was quick to point out.

"Oh yes, your new shoes look great too."

"I go scoo now, kay?"

"It's still too early yet, Jade. We've got another hour before we have to leave. You have lots of time, so why don't you go into the bathroom, wash up, brush your teeth, and brush your hair."

"Did it weddy, Gayo."

Jade went into the kitchen and sat on the small bench, staring at the digital clock. She asked, "What nummers?"

"Eight-three-zero," I replied.

At eight-thirty sharp, Jade leaped up from the bench.

"Time fer scoo," she shouted. "Wet's go!"

We were no sooner out the front door, when I snapped a photo of Jade and she tripped on the sidewalk, scraping her knee. She quickly got up from the pavement and was about to cry, when she must have realized that it was too important a day for tears. With a crack in her voice, she said, "Wet's go, Mommy. No be wate."

Being the first day of school, most mothers remained with their child in the classroom for the first half hour. Although Jade seemed to be a little shy among all these new faces, as soon as she spotted Miss Klein in the crowded room, she went over to greet her by name. "She already remembers the teacher's name," one parent remarked. Little did she know that Jade had practised it all summer.

I followed Jade over to the chalkboard where she started to scribble some letters. I crouched down to her level in order to have a little chat with her, hopefully easing any tension she might have.

"Jade," I began, "this is your new class, and all of the kids are here for the very first time, just like you. After a while, everybody is going to know one another and become friends. You also have to work while you're here, but you love arts and crafts and stories, right?"

In a hushed voice, Jade replied, "Yeah, Mommy, I wike it. You go home now, kay?"

"Fine, Jade. I'll come back for you at lunch time."

After only one week, Jade's integration into the kindergarten was proving to be successful. She loved going to school, and each morning as she arrived at the schoolyard, she was greeted by most of her classmates. The only complaint Jade seemed to have was that two and a half hours of school wasn't enough for her. Each day after lunch, she'd ask to return to school.

About a week later, Jade began participating in an afternoon preschool program that was held every day at this same school. For Jade, this program was like taking a break. After a morning of instruction, she had the opportunity to spend a relaxing afternoon, playing and socializing with another group of children, many of whom she had already befriended through summer day camp.

When meeting Jade after kindergarten class each morning, I asked the teacher how things were going. "Fine," Miss Klein answered. "No problem."

But somehow I found it difficult to believe. This integration program was a brand new experience for everyone. How could everything be running so smoothly, so quickly? I had been expecting at least some adjustments on the teacher's part, as well as on that of Jade and the other kindergarten students.

About two weeks later, Miss Klein requested that I spend some time in the classroom. Uh-oh, here it comes, I thought. Things mustn't be running so smoothly after all.

While the children were seated in a circle on the floor during show-and-tell, I sat at the back of the classroom, observing. But Jade didn't wander off from the group, as I might have expected, seeking other things to do. So much for her supposed shorter attention span.

Later, the group followed the teacher to the chalkboard where they were given illustrations concerning spatial concepts. Each child, including Jade, was called upon to contribute his or her own ideas. Jade took the class work quite seriously and was very attentive, even more so than some of the other pupils. Then again, with all of Jade's early years of stimulation programs, she was practically trained to listen and apply herself.

The class was given a simple assignment based on the subject that had been discussed earlier on. Each child returned to his or her individual desk, was handed a stencilled sheet, and got to work. It was at this time that Jade required one-on-one instruction. Linda, the special education teacher, entered the classroom, sat down at the reserved desk next to Jade's and proceeded to help. This was wonderful, I thought. No disruption whatsoever. It seemed so normal and natural for an assistant to casually join in the classroom work at some point during the morning.

When the pupils recessed for a snack, Miss Klein came over to me. "Now that I've gotten to know Jade better," she explained, "I can clue into areas where she requires extra help, and sometimes all that's required is an extra few minutes of explanation. The timing arrangement I have with the special-ed teacher is working out perfectly. When Linda is not here helping Jade, she is assisting another student in another class."

"What about Jade's language?" I enquired. "Do you have any trouble understanding her?"

"Yes, as a matter of fact, I do," she said. "Sometimes Jade says things that are not very clear to me, but her classmates seem to understand her." She smiled and added, "When Jade has trouble making herself understood, she looks to another child for assistance, or shall I say, a translation. I'm so pleased to have Jade in my class and, as you can see, she is well-liked and accepted by her peers. I know you've been worried, so I wanted you to see for yourself how things are progressing. I'm glad you came into the classroom to observe. Now you can rest assured that Jade is doing well, and I've come to better understand that Jade really isn't much different from the other children."

I was so relieved and elated that I almost wanted to kiss the teacher. I then spoke with the school principal, who said, "The kindergarten teacher, as well as the first and second grade teachers of the other special pupils, are very happy that things are running so smoothly. And I'm very pleased with our three special students."

Since class was almost over, rather than returning home, I went downstairs and stood by the schoolyard door to wait for Jade.

Miss Klein led the class through the corridor and then down the stairs to the exit. Jade usually walked by Miss Klein's side at the front of the line, although on a couple of occasions, she lagged behind, walking at a much slower pace. There were a few children, however, who seemed to be on guard for Jade and let the teacher know. "Wait up, Miss Klein, wait up for Jade."

This truly was an ideal education, I thought, for everyone. Children as young as five years of age were learning patience, tolerance and, best of all, gaining firsthand knowledge about children with special needs.

After school hours, Jade was happy to see her friends at the park, and it was obvious that those feelings were mutual. There was only one thing that she didn't particularly favour: her small size seemed to make some kids over-protective of her, and she just wanted to be an equal part of the gang. She'd often pull away when another child wanted to hug her or take her by the hand. Although she must have known that these intentions were kind, she insisted: "No touch hand. I a big girl."

Both Jade and I had certain adjustments to make—lunch invitations, for example. On several occasions, one of Jade's classmates, Pamela, had invited Jade to lunch, but Jade declined each time. Neither of us was used to this—it was too "normal." Jade had never before had the opportunity to socialize without my having to make the arrangement first. It was as though I, too, had to be integrated into normal society.

I later spoke with Pamela's mother, who mentioned that her daughter was very eager to have Jade come over to their house to play. "Pam just adores Jade," she said, "and she wants to become closer friends with her."

Jade accepted Pamela's invitation the following week, though both of us were still trying to get used to this new social life. It was all so normal, and I was deeply touched.

CHAPTER THIRTEEN

On Friday, September 20, when Jade arrived home from her afternoon program, she headed directly for the living room couch. She was extremely tired and breathed heavily with a slight cough; there was a bluish colouring to her lips and nails.

Since her regular pediatrician was away on holiday, I brought her to a local clinic, where I was informed that she had a touch of bronchitis. Antibiotics were prescribed, and I was told that she should feel a lot better within a few days.

Three days went by, but there was no change. Jade hadn't any appetite. She became extremely weak, had constant fevers, and was uninterested in anything but sleep. I took her to the regular pediatrician, who was back from vacation by then, and her diagnosis was also "bronchitis." She said that Jade's loss of appetite and her listlessness were side effects of the antibiotics and that I should let the medication run its course.

On the doctor's advice, I made sure that Jade finished the antibiotics. And there were changes in her health—but changes for the worse. She was now sleeping twenty-four hours a day, only waking for twenty-minute intervals, at which time I tried to spoon-feed her with applesauce or some warm soup, along with some juice and water to keep her hydrated. Her breathing became more difficult, and she was coughing incessantly.

Exactly seven days after the onset of this illness, I determined that Jade's condition must be something more than bronchitis. I brought her to the hospital where she had x-rays and culture tests.

Although frail, Jade still managed to put up a strong fight.

Two nurses, an intern, and I tried to restrain her while an intravenous tube was being attached to her left hand. I couldn't bear it—the screaming, the crying, the kicking, the helplessness. I broke down and started to cry myself. My legs were shaking, and I felt faint.

Later, while seated outside one of the examination rooms with Jade curled up on my lap, I noticed two doctors examining someone's x-ray as they held it up to the light. They then looked over at me. One of the doctors approached me and said that Cardiology's resident doctor was now being called in to examine Jade.

I had a headache that seemed to be getting stronger by the second, and my heart was pounding faster now. After what seemed like an eternity, I was greeted by Dr. Brian Hanna. I was asked to carry Jade into the examination room once again. She started to cry, her legs wrapped tightly around my waist and her arms wound around my neck. The doctor was very gentle, as he explained to Jade that he was just going to do a very small examination that won't hurt at all, and that when he was done, she could have the stethoscope to listen to her own heart. Jade still wasn't cooperative, but she was a lot calmer.

After this second examination was over, I was shown Jade's chest x-ray. Dr. Hanna pointed out the heavily clouded areas. "Your daughter has pneumonia," he said. "There's a large amount of fluid in her lungs, and her heart, beating at such a fast rate, is working too hard. Your daughter is experiencing heart failure and we will be giving her digoxin, a heart drug to help slow the heart rate. In addition, she will be given diuretics, which will help eliminate, by urinating, some of the fluid in her lungs. Along with taking antibiotics, which will be administered intravenously, Jade will be placed in an oxygen tent that will help to ease her breathing. I will contact the cardiology ward where she can be admitted right away, and it'll probably be a few days before she is strong enough to recuperate at home."

When I returned home about midnight, I collapsed onto the couch. In my mind, I kept picturing Jade's helpless state, her fighting with the doctors, and the hurt she must have felt when I

134

couldn't help her.

It was a nightmarish feeling, though not the first, of coming home from the hospital—alone. My heart just ached for Jade as I went into her bedroom. I laid in her bed holding Jo-Jo, her favourite doll.

I was not a very religious person, at least not as religious as my father would have liked me to be, since I didn't attend church regularly. But although I often had doubts about God, I figured I had nothing to lose at this point in trying to pray. There was no one person in this world who could possibly help me, so I had to force myself to believe that there really was a God. During my most difficult, trying times, I had no choice but to believe that there was someone out there listening to me and caring about me. So I prayed like I never prayed before.

By 6 A.M. I had showered, dressed, gathered some of Jade's belongings and returned to the hospital. I wanted to be there before Jade awoke that morning.

Over the next few days, Jade continued to be listless; the fevers persisted, and she hadn't any appetite.

I met with Jade's regular cardiologist, Dr. Gibbons, in his office. "First of all," he said, "I want you to know that I think you've been doing a wonderful job with Jade." He continued, "As you know, we've been treating her with antibiotics, but she hasn't been responding to them, and we'll just have to keep trying different kinds in hopes that one of them will cure her of whatever virus she has contracted. The fevers are still occurring, mainly at night, and they'll probably continue until we find the right antibiotic. We've taken further x-rays and, because of the diuretics, some of the fluid in Jade's lungs has been eliminated. Unfortunately, every time Jade gets ill, it creates further wear and tear on her heart."

I braced myself, trying very hard to hold back the tears, waiting for the worst.

"But I'm optimistic," the doctor said. "Jade has never

before required any heart medication; she has always been very strong and active. But I am now going to prescribe a heart drug that should be given to her regularly. It'll help slow down the heart rate, easing some of the pressure, so that her heart will not have to work so hard. With her heart beating at an easier pace, it should also help to build her resistance. I have a feeling that once Jade combats this illness, with this heart medication, she may be even better than she was before. We'll give it a few more days and monitor her response to the treatment. Then hopefully, she'll soon be able to return home to recuperate."

As I headed up to the seventh floor to Jade's room, which she shared with three other youngsters, I felt a tremendous sense of relief. Jade's going to get better, I thought, better than she's ever been.

With tears streaming down her face, Jade was sitting up in her bed, watching for me through the room's large windowpane.

I held her in my arms, stroking her hair and kissing her face. "The doctor told me, Jade, that you're going to get better real soon. Isn't that good news?"

"Go home now, Mommy," she cried.

"Yes, darling, probably in a few days. And we're going to have a little party just for you. And with prizes too."

Nothing seemed to interest Jade, though. She just wanted to get out of this place, and I certainly couldn't blame her for that.

"Guess what?" I said.

"What?" Finally, a sign of interest.

"Andrew is coming here later, and he has a surprise for you."

"Pize?" Jade asked with a little more interest.

"Yes, sweetheart, Andrew wants to visit you and give you a nice present."

"Ah, nice Andu," she said.

A physiotherapist then entered the room. "It's time for us to play a game now, Jade. I have something I think you're going to like, but first we have to do some exercises."

Jade refused to let this woman touch her, but by now, I

knew what was required.

"Mommy do it," Jade demanded.

I proceeded with the clapping. Jade wasn't too keen on this, preferring a back massage, but the clapping on her chest and sides helped to loosen the mucus.

The therapist then handed Jade a bottle of bubbles. She refused to accept it, although once the therapist left the room, she decided that she'd like to blow bubbles after all. She even smiled. God, it'd been so long since I've seen her smile!

A nurse then walked in. "Time to take your temperature, Jade."

Jade's smile quickly vanished. By now she knew that arguing served no purpose and gave in, but under one condition, which she made perfectly clear to the nursing staff. "Mommy do it, no you!"

At least there was something that made me feel useful these days. At least Jade trusted me. I had been so worried that she would lose her trust in me, because I was the one who brought her for x-rays; I was the one who brought her for blood tests; and I was the one who brought her to the hospital in the first place.

Dr. Hanna then came in to see how we were doing. He struck me as a very kind, gentle person, since he would never *force* Jade to cooperate; instead, he took the time to comfort her with gentle, reassuring words. There was a human side to this doctor that I didn't see in the others. He asked me a lot of questions about Jade, about her school, about her interests, and I never got the feeling that he was just making small talk; I got the feeling that he was genuinely interested in knowing Jade as a person and not just as a patient. Also, when he looked at me, it wasn't a look of pity, but rather, if I'm not mistaken, it was a look of admiration. But for what, I didn't know.

After eating a little soup and drinking some juice, Jade napped for almost three hours. When she awoke, Andrew was sitting in an armchair beside her bed, but Jade seemed uninterested in seeing anyone except me. Not her grandparents, aunts, or uncles—no one. She silently observed Andrew as he assembled a cardboard farmhouse on her food tray.

A nurse then walked in with Jade's medication. "It's time for your medicine now, Jade."

"Oh no," she whimpered, "no gen."

From the window I had been observing Jade and Andrew—and the nurse. The nurse! I promptly dashed into the room to take my guarded position next to Jade.

With relief, Jade looked at me, then glared at the nurse. "Mommy gimme it, no you!" She took the medicine, then managed a tiny smile as she pointed to her farmhouse. "Wook," she said, "Andu gimme pize."

"Oh, Jade, it's beautiful. Such nice, colourful farm animals too. Why don't the three of us play with it now?"

She shrugged her shoulders, saying, "No, I tire. You and Andu pay wif animos."

She rested her head against the pillow, fighting to keep her eyes open but fell asleep.

The following morning, I overslept. I didn't arrive at the hospital until after ten o'clock. Jade, I learned, had been given more blood tests that morning and a heart ultrasound.

"The doctor will be advising you later," one nurse said to me.

"Please," I emphasized, "I would appreciate it if any tests could be taken only when I'm present. Jade is much more cooperative when I am with her, and she needs me by her side."

"I'm aware of your request," the nurse replied. "However, certain tests have to be done at certain times." She went on, "By the way, Jade isn't in her room right now. She was brought to the playroom to watch television."

I walked into the playroom to find two small children contentedly playing some games with one of the hospital's volunteers. Jade was seated on a small rocking chair, her head resting on the arm of the chair. I called out to her. As she raised her head, tears were coursing down her cheeks. She then managed a tiny smile. "Oh Mommy," she cried as she reached out her arms to me, "You come bissit me." The tears in Jade's eyes brought tears to my eyes, and I just wanted us to get the hell out of here, away from this painful place.

"I love you so much, Jade. You know that, eh?"

"Yeah, Mommy, I wuv you," she said as she clung to me. I asked if she wanted to play with some puzzles.

"No," she replied wearily, "I too tire."

Jade clung to me tighter, not wanting me to put her down. "Guess what?" I said. "Joan is coming to visit you today."

Jade eyes instantly lit up. "Joan coming bissit me?"

"Yes, darling, Joan is coming!"

"Oh goody. Hank you. Oh gweat!"

Jade started to giggle as I carried her back to her room.

Jade was so happy to see Joan, ate all of her lunch, then showed some interest in the story that Joan was reading to her.

That afternoon I saw the cardiologist. During his rounds, he came to see me at Jade's bedside and advised me of the morning's test results. I was told that the antibiotics hadn't been effective, and that the morning's heart ultrasound showed a significant amount of fluid in the lining of Jade's heart. "The medical term used," he said, "is pericarditis—an infection of the lining of the heart. Among the probable causes are a cold or the flu, which are caused by viruses." He added, "If I can have your permission, Gail, I would like to remove as much of the fluid as possible. The fluid can be extracted with a fine needle and the only treatment necessary after that would be aspirin or acetaminophen."

I was so relieved that there was finally a solution, but I was also scared. The few days that Jade was expected to stay in the hospital turned into fifteen. Her morale was so low that I just didn't know how much more she, or I, could take of this.

I met with two resident doctors as they were doing their rounds. "It's no wonder Jade is so listless with all that weight around her heart," one of them said. "Dr. Gibbons is very adept in his work, and once the fluid has been removed, Jade will soon pick up and be on the road to recovery," they assured me.

After Jade had been sedated, two nurses wheeled her bed to another ward, where Dr. Gibbons was to remove the fluid.

It's not surgery, I kept reminding myself. The doctor

knows what he's doing. I had this gnawing feeling in my stomach, unable to bring myself to leave Jade's hospital room. Silently I prayed, staring into the spot where Jade's bed had been. I then started to cry as I thought of all the prayers that went unanswered. I found myself starting to get uptight and angry that Jade, one of the most loving people in this world, had to go through all this. Why, God? Why Jade?

I took Jade's get-well cards from the windowsill and started to read them. They were from her teachers and classmates of both morning and afternoon classes. I thought about what the special education teacher had told me during a recent telephone conversation:

"The children miss Jade very much and are constantly asking about her. One of the children started to weep when she learned that Jade was in the hospital. We think and talk about her everyday, and the children have been reassured that Jade will be returning to class just as soon as she's feeling better."

As I placed the cards back onto the windowsill, a pretty girl, about fifteen, walked into the room. With a look of uncertainty, she asked, "Are you Jade's mother?"

I nodded. Although she looked very familiar, the name didn't click.

"Well, I don't know if you remember me, but I'm Miranda. Two summers ago, I was a camp counsellor-in-training. Anyway, I just heard from a neighbour that Jade was in the hospital, and I wanted to visit her."

Puzzled, looking at the vacant space where Jade's bed must have been, Miranda quietly asked, "Where is she?"

I explained briefly what was happening. Miranda seemed so genuinely relieved when I told her that once the fluid was removed, Jade would recover soon afterward.

"Thank goodness," she said, "I was really worried about her."

As I thanked Miranda for her thoughtful visit, she handed me a nicely wrapped gift.

"I'd better get back to school now," she said, "but please give this to Jade. It's a colouring book and some crayons."

140

Jade was still in a sound sleep when she was returned to the room. "Everything went well," I was told by one of the doctors. "A large amount of fluid had been extracted. With all that extra pressure removed, there should now be a noticeable improvement."

Later, the cardiologist advised me that Jade should be able to return home within a few days to recuperate. "We'll do another ultrasound in a couple of days," he said, "just to confirm that most of the fluid has been removed. You will then be shown by the nurses how to administer the exact dosages of heart medication that will be prescribed for Jade."

With tremendous relief and happiness I told everyone the great news. Jade would be coming home soon.

Over the next two days, I waited patiently for Jade to wake up, but she slept most of the time, waking only for fifteen minute intervals, usually to be given her medication. I sat there day and night, just waiting and hoping that she'd wake up and want to play, or at least talk. But she wouldn't, or couldn't, talk and simply nodded her head *yes* or *no*.

The effects of the sedation were slowly wearing off, when Jade at last sat up in bed. She was so obviously frustrated, as doctors and nurses constantly probed at her; pricked her fingers and toes for blood cultures; took her temperature, x-rays, and ultrasounds; and administered medication. It's no wonder that she rebelled in probably the only way she knew. After deliberately knocking the small plastic cup of medication from the nurse's hand, when given the replacement dose, Jade spat it on the floor.

Good for you, Jade, I thought. Let it out. You have every right to rebel. I knew, of course, that this was not the best way to rebel, but I totally understood her frustration.

Because I wanted to avoid Jade's being alone during her waking hours, Joan obligingly filled in for me whenever she was needed. It was such a good feeling to know that there was at least one other person in this world with whom Jade felt secure.

141

Jade's appetite had increased slightly and once again she had a good, healthy complexion. She stayed awake for about half-hour intervals now, but she wouldn't talk to anyone—not even to me. I'd gently rub her back until she fell asleep again.

One day, after waking up from one of these long naps, Jade's eyes popped open with curiosity when she noticed a large parcel at the foot of her bed.

"What's dat?" she asked.

"I don't know, Jade. A nurse delivered it while you were asleep, telling me that someone brought it to the hospital for you. I wonder what it is."

"I open it?" she asked.

"Of course, Jade, it's for you. Look, the bag has your name on it."

Suddenly, a big happy smile came to Jade's face as she pulled the large, plastic pumpkin from the bag.

"A pumkin!" she exclaimed. "It's Hoween time?"

"Look, Jade," I said, "there's a card. It's from Pamela! Oh, Pamela is such a sweetheart, isn't she?"

"Yeah, Pam's cute; Pam my fend."

Jade eagerly sorted through all the little surprises in the pumpkin: markers, stickers, a pad of note paper, a Care Bear drinking cup, and a few little Halloween treats. The perfect medicine. Something to take her mind off this place, if only for a while, and to remind her of the fun that awaited on Halloween.

As Jade and I were drawing pictures of pumpkins and ghosts, a nurse walked in and asked me to bring Jade downstairs for another ultrasound.

Jade, gathering and clinging onto her markers and papers, understood every word. "No," she insisted, "I say here!"

"Jade," I explained, "this might be the very last test." And I really hoped and expected that it would be just a confirmation that all of the fluid had been removed, and that everything would be fine now.

Later, the cardiologist came to see me in Jade's room. "I regret to tell you," he said, "that the fluid that was removed the other day has now re-accumulated. Should the fluid be removed again, there's no guarantee that it will not return. The only thing we can do now is continue treating Jade with steady doses of aspirin, which is the only known treatment for pericarditis. Eliminating the fluid may be a very slow process, but we'll just have to be patient."

When the doctor left, I was holding Jade tightly for comfort. I was scared and lost at this turn of events and didn't quite know what to do. What really frightened me was that I couldn't help Jade. My body was frozen. I couldn't cry, for the tears had frozen within me.

That's it, I decided, we're going home. I can't tolerate this place any longer.

CHAPTER FOURTEEN

I did my best to convince the doctors that Jade would, in all probability, recuperate more quickly at home. "I'm positive that once Jade is in her own familiar surroundings, she'll begin to eat better, and her morale will be restored." To my relief, they agreed. They were only too well aware that Jade was losing far too much weight, and her exceedingly low spirits weren't helping matters.

I was given strict, detailed instructions as far as Jade's medication was concerned and was also put in touch with the cardiology nurse, Connie, who was to keep daily contact with me.

The following day, as Jade awoke from her nap, her eyes lit up and a smile lit up on her face. There, neatly laid out on her bed, were her clothes and her jacket. Andrew and I stood by, anticipating her response.

Then, with a look of disbelief, Jade stared at us both. "Go home now?" she asked.

"Yes, my darling," I was so happy to say, "today you are going home."

Excited, Jade grabbed her jacket and attempted to put it on quickly.

"Slow down, Jade," Andrew said. "You have to put your clothes on first."

When Jade was fully dressed, she hurriedly went over to a couple of nurses at the nursing station. "I go home now!" she exclaimed. "Goo-bye eva-body."

While Andrew and I were double-checking that we had all of Jade's belongings, Jade was heading down the corridor to the elevator.

As Andrew carried Jade up the stairs to our flat, Jade gave him a big hug. "I happy, Andu! My home!"

"We're all so happy, Jade. We missed you so much, and I'll bet you're anxious to play with all your toys again."

After taking a long look in every room, absorbing all she had missed, Jade went into her bedroom. She went from playing with her musical organ, to her dolls, to her trucks, and then to her record player.

It must have then occurred to Jade that while coming up the stairwell to our house, she noticed some Halloween decorations hanging on the walls. She left her room, opened the front door, then motioned for me to join her.

"Hoween, Mommy? I go twick-o-tweet?"

"Yes, Jade, that's right. Next week it'll be Halloween, and Andrew and I are going to take you out."

"Oh boy! You and me and Andu."

The three of us spent the next little while drawing Halloween pictures, then hanging the pictures on the walls.

After a light supper, Jade had a warm bath while I read to her. She enjoyed listening to "The King's Birthday," a simple story from which she had memorized most of the words.

When Jade went to bed she God-blessed Halloween, then fell asleep.

About three hours later I looked in on her. She was sleeping so peacefully and had such a wonderful day that I hated to wake her, but it was time for her medication.

"Oh no, Mommy," she whined wearily.

"It's okay, Jade, just take this and then you can go back to sleep."

Deeply relieved to have her back home again, back in her own bed, I kissed her beautiful face, then stroked her hair.

Several hours later, I again had to wake her. It was time to take some more aspirin. I felt like such a cruel mother. Just when Jade thought she was free from having to take any more medicine, I had to insist on her taking more.

I hadn't slept much of that first night that Jade was back,

145

as I was worried that I mightn't remember to give her the proper medication at the proper time. Although I had a written schedule, I especially worried about the heart drug, digoxin, as I knew how dangerous this drug was if administered in an incorrect dosage. I then decided to set my alarm clock one hour prior to giving this drug in the morning, ensuring that I was fully awake before taking any measurements.

As promised, Andrew and I took Jade trick-or-treating on Halloween night, and because Jade hadn't fully regained her strength, Andrew carried her from door to door, and we kept our outing to a maximum forty-five minutes.

Over the next week Jade did fairly well; her appetite improved and she slowly got back to some of the activities she enjoyed.

A few of my friends came by with their children to visit, but their stays were brief, as Jade still required a lot of rest.

Jade napped for a couple of hours each morning and afternoon, then went to bed by seven o'clock each night. On some nights, she was keen enough to listen to stories. She requested two books in particular, which were the Christian storybooks I gave her while she was in the hospital. It was very light reading in easy-to-understand verse. Although Jade learned at a very early age about Jesus, I didn't know how much she could understand. Exactly what prayers meant to her, I also didn't know. All I knew was that she loved to say them.

Jade listened to the stories intently. It was as though the author was speaking to her directly about love, respect, forgiveness, and kindness. Through the use of simple terms, Jade was now learning more about Jesus' love, that He created the world and everybody in it. As she sat in bed, she kept nodding her head, wanting to hear more, devouring each word as it was read.

We returned to the hospital for Jade's cardiology appointment. After a heart ultrasound was taken, I was informed that there hadn't been any significant change. Only a small amount of the fluid around the heart had been eliminated. "It's a slow process," the doctor explained, "and I realize it's upsetting for you, but you'll just have to be patient." He paused. "Although the improvement has been minimal, there has been some improvement and, little by little, the fluid will be eliminated."

Each morning over the next two weeks, I took Jade out for a walk in her stroller. It was such a beautiful neighbourhood with lots of shady trees and huge, old, character houses.

When we arrived at the corner of our street, Jade excitedly greeted the school's crossing guard. "Hi, coss god," she said and laughed. The crossing guard was always very friendly with Jade and spent a few minutes to chat.

"My scoo," Jade exclaimed as she pointed it out to me. "Wanna go at scoo."

It would have broken my heart to tell Jade that she wasn't well enough to return to school yet, so I lied.

"Jade," I explained, "there are no kindergarten classes this week because of holidays, but I think classes will probably start again next week."

Disappointed, she said, "Ah, mayme nex week."

After giving it a great deal of thought, I consulted with the cardiology nurse. She agreed that Jade's return to school mightn't be a bad idea, at least for part of the morning.

I then arranged with the teachers to have Jade spend an hour in class each morning, increasing the duration of time as Jade's health improved.

Jade's classmates were delighted to see her and came running to greet her when she arrived. There were a lot of happy voices exclaiming, "She's here! Jade's back!"

Jade's special buddy, Pam, was so happy to learn of Jade's return that she actually started to cry.

An hour of schoolwork was about all Jade could handle for the time being, but she seemed content with the routine, and she was given the choice each morning as to whether or not she wanted to go to school.

Because Jade was still physically weak, I brought her to school about twenty minutes after class started, carried her up the stairs to the second floor, then returned an hour later to carry her back down.

It was nice to hear Jade talking about school once again, and she loved to bring back some homework.

One morning, a week after Jade's return to school, I received a call from Linda, the special-ed teacher. She said, "The kindergarten teacher is very concerned about Jade. We don't think she's feeling well. She's extremely tired, and her breathing is very rapid."

Within ten minutes, I was at the school and went into the classroom. The children were sitting in a circle around Miss Klein's chair, while she was reading a story. Jade was seated on her lap, her head resting on the teacher's shoulder.

Miss Klein carried Jade over to me and, in a sympathetic voice, said, "I'm really worried about her. Her breathing is very rapid, and when I picked her up she just about fell asleep on me."

I thanked Miss Klein for advising me of this right away, dressed Jade in her snowsuit, and was escorted home by Linda.

After notifying Connie, the cardiology nurse, I brought Jade to the hospital. As the taxi pulled up at the emergency entrance Jade cried, "No Mommy! No Hoppito! No Mommy!"

My stomach was tied up in knots, and I just wanted to scream. I wanted to yell out, "No, God, we've had enough of this! When are you going to give us a break?"

There had been more fluid buildup. "What we can do," Dr. Hanna said, "is give Jade some Lasix, a highly effective diuretic, right here and now. It'll help get rid of that excess fluid. In the meantime, I'd advise that you keep her home from school, let her get lots of rest, and advise Connie every day how things are going."

I was slow in dressing Jade as I tried to think of questions to ask.

The doctor looked at me, "You do have a choice," he said. "Jade can either be admitted to the cardiology ward for a day or two, or she can go home and be given the same treatment

148

under your care."

Without hesitation, I replied, "Of course, I'd prefer to take care of her myself."

Over the next week Jade's appetite decreased and she was now sleeping for most of the day and night.

One night I was awakened by loud screams. I ran into Jade's room and saw her sitting up in bed, her arms folded around her stomach. She started to scream again. I massaged her stomach, trying to comfort her as she cried, "Tummy hutts!" She refused to lie down.

I was trying to understand what was happening, and for one terrifying moment, I thought: maybe this is it. Maybe this is the tragic end. I cried and the miseries took over. Suddenly there was a hand on my face and a voice saying, "Mommy, why cying?"

"Oh, Jade, I'm sorry," I said. "It's just that my stomach hurts, too." As I reached for a Kleenex from the night-stand, I added, "But I'm okay now. I feel better. Are you okay?"

"Yeah, Mommy. Touch my face."

I stroked Jade's soft, warm face until we both fell asleep.

I called Dr. Hanna the next morning. After I informed him about the events of the previous night, his advice was: "If Jade is uncomfortable lying down, I suggest that you prop two or three pillows at her back. What is happening is that when Jade is in a horizontal position, the fluid from her tissues is accumulating around her heart thus causing the chest pains."

"Well, what can I do about it? How can I stop the pain?"

"You can't," the doctor replied. "You are doing everything you can do for her right now. Along with giving Jade the medication, just try to keep her as comfortable as possible. We've just got to hope that she beats this terrible virus, and if we could do more, we would be doing it."

Jade slept for most of that day and didn't experience any pain that night, but on the following night the chest pains recurred. I raced into her room as soon as the screaming started. Her pillows were propped up as they had been all day. I held her in my arms for the entire night, while she slept intermittently—crying for a few minutes, then sleeping for a few more. I was

149

losing hope. What if she never gets better? As I lay awake, holding Jade in my arms, I prayed:

"Lord, she is peaceful now. If it is Your intention to take my baby away from me, do it now, right at this very moment while I am with her and she feels my warmth and my love. Please, Lord, take her before she awakens with more pain. You, more than anyone, should know that Jade doesn't deserve all this suffering. And please, Lord, if You do decide to take her from me, give her all Your love, and I'm trusting You to take good care of her. I'm ready now, Lord, and please remember that I'm trusting You with my baby."

I was trying to make some sort of sense out of that awful and beautiful moment when Jade woke up. More pain. When the crying stopped and she fell back to sleep, I prayed again, but this time I was angry.

"Lord, how could You do this to us? Please—if it is not Your will to take Jade, then I beg You to please make her better. Make the pain go away! Give Jade a brand new chance at life. She needs me, Lord, and You know how much I need her. You've blessed me with this special child, enriching my life, and now You are making us so miserable. Why are You doing this to us?"

The days were excruciatingly long. Jade slept most of the time while I dragged my feet about the house. Out of boredom I tried reading novels, but no stories were interesting enough. I tried cooking, but no food tasted good enough. I tried watching television, but the images were unclear, and the sound was muffled. There was only so much cleaning a house required, and the plants were over-watered. What next? I simply waited for Jade to wake up for a while so I could make her more comfortable, try to feed her, give her some juice, talk to her, hold her, tell her how much I love her, then go to another room to cry while she slept again.

Meantime, there was no money coming in. I was forced to leave my evening job to be home with Jade. Being self-employed, I was billing the company monthly, but was ineligible for unemployment insurance. While Andrew and a couple of my brothers helped with the rent and other expenses during this time, no matter how extenuating the circumstances, it was still an incredible blow to my pride to accept money from anyone. A bigger blow, however, was going to the Welfare Bureau to apply for social assistance. The choice of avoiding *charity* after all these years was no longer an option. More humiliating than asking for a handout was having to claim that I didn't know who the biological father was, otherwise I'd have been forced to seek a lawyer to fight for child support. It was a fight I wasn't prepared to undertake, not now, not ever.

Every night was a sleepless night. On the nights that Jade did sleep comfortably, I stayed awake, almost anticipating a scream. One evening, determined to catch up on some sleep, I retired early. I felt emotionally drained and must have fallen asleep just seconds after my head touched the pillow. On this particular night, because I was so determined to get some sleep, I had kept my door completely closed, since I'd always run to Jade at her slightest stir. Jade then let out a loud scream. Startled, I jumped out of bed and made a dash to her room. I smashed into the door, jabbing the door knob into my hip. I was so tired and angry that with all the firmness and authority I could manage, I yelled, "Jade, stop it! Stop it now! Go to sleep! No more screaming!" I thought the whole neighbourhood must have heard me.

Jade was silent for a moment. Then I heard her crying quietly. Oh my God! My poor baby! How could I yell at her when she's in such pain? It's not her fault—God knows it's not her fault.

I went into Jade's room to comfort her. As I turned on the night-light, I saw tears steaming down her face.

"I sowee, Mommy," she sobbed.

Trying very hard to hide my own tears, I said, "Oh, Jade, I'm sorry too. You're such a sweet, beautiful angel, and I'm so sorry that I yelled at you. It's not your fault. It's mine. I only yelled because I had a little accident."

She just looked at me, waiting for an explanation.

"I bumped into my bedroom door," I explained, "and it

hurt. That's why I got angry. I'm not angry at you; I'm angry at me." I forced a laugh. "Silly Mommy, eh?"

"Yeah, you siddy, Mommy," though without an accompanying smile, her words were less than convincing.

That night turned out to be like many of the others: agonizing moments of pain and quiet intermissions of sleep.

The next morning I called Dr. Hanna. "Jade's in such pain," I said. "You *must* be able to do something."

He advised me to admit Jade to the hospital for a couple of days in order to run some tests and, if so required, he would make changes to her medication.

While Jade slept, I gathered some of her belongings: her two Barbie dolls, her favourite rag doll, her photo album, some colouring books and crayons.

I dreaded the thought of re-admitting Jade to the hospital. It is really going to crush her, I worried. And it is really going to crush me. I didn't know if either of us could handle it again.

At noon, Evy picked us up and drove us to the hospital. Jade was so sleepy that she hadn't noticed where we were until we arrived at the admitting office. She didn't put up a fight this time. I lifted her onto a wheelchair, and we proceeded to the elevator. I was amazed. Jade hadn't complained. She relayed a quiet "Hello" to the nurses as we entered the cardiology ward.

I brought Jade to her bed. No arguments whatsoever. In fact, she seemed to be quite relaxed, smiling whenever she saw a familiar face. It was as though, as one nurse put it, "She now realizes that this is the place to be helped when you're sick."

Five minutes later, Jade stated that she was hungry. While I went to the kitchen at the end of the corridor to prepare a sandwich, Jade warmed up to Evy, showing her the prized pictures in her photo album.

Later, she had her finger pricked for a blood culture test. Because she seemed to scream louder at the sight of the band-aid, I put a couple on my own fingers. All of a sudden, the band-aid didn't seem like such a horrible thing. Jade unwrapped a few, sticking them on her doll, Jo-Jo.

"Same," she said.

"Yes, Jade. Now we're all the same."

At about nine o'clock that night, I left for home. I knew that I was permitted to rest on a cot in the playroom down the hall from Jade's room, but I also knew that it was a place that I couldn't actually sleep, for all the clattering I would hear. On the other hand, I couldn't sleep at home either. Somehow my worries and fears would always hit me the hardest in the middle of the night. It was a time when I most needed to be assured that Jade was all right.

The following morning when I arrived at the hospital, Jade was sitting on Joan's lap, talking and laughing with her. Thank goodness for Joan.

I was informed by a nurse that after an injection of Lasix, Jade slept soundly the whole night through.

That afternoon, Dr. Gibbons came to see me. I was lying beside Jade in her bed, expecting some hopeful, good news. He began, "After studying the results of Jade's latest tests, what I have to tell you isn't good." My whole body tensed up, and I tried to say something to stop him from continuing, but nothing came.

He went on, "There has been serious deterioration of Jade's heart, and as you know, there is nothing we can do about it. We can't cure Jade's heart defect, but we've tried everything to help cure her from this virus in order to prevent further deterioration. Jade hasn't been able to beat this virus, and at this point, I don't expect she'll get any better. Her condition will likely worsen as time goes on. All we can do now is to continue with the medication to help relieve the pain and try to make her as comfortable as possible. I think you should prepare yourself . . . "

At this excruciating moment, I was no longer able to see the doctor for the tears that were clouding my vision; nor was I able to hear whatever else he had to say. I was numb. He left the room, and I found myself cradling Jade in my arms, wanting to be cradled myself.

Jade saw the hurt in my eyes. Touching my face, she

153

started to cry. "Aah, no sad, Mommy, kay? Matta, Mommy? Matta?"

I couldn't answer her. "Jade," I finally mustered, "do you want to play with some puzzles?" She hesitated, then shook her head. We went into the playroom, but I simply couldn't concentrate on playing.

My thoughts were scared and angry. How dare he drop a bomb on me like that—without even a warning! How dare he talk about Jade's condition, saying that she will *never* get better—in Jade's very presence! Did he think that Jade was too retarded to understand?

Jade put a puzzle piece in my hand, then guided my hand to the appropriate space. "I'm sorry, Jade, I'm not doing too well with this, am I?"

"Dat's kay, Mommy, I'm show you."

Jade continued talking to me, but I couldn't really hear what she was saying. All I could hear, over and over again, was: "Prepare yourself."

Prepare myself for what? Prepare myself for more unbearable suffering? Prepare myself for Jade's death? Prepare myself for life after Jade? God, I just can't do it. Don't You do this to me, or I'll hate You forever!

I felt weak and hot. It was so freaking hot in this place!

I took Jade from the small chair, held her tightly, then buried my face in her neck and started to cry. Damn it! That was all Jade needed now! I had to find a way to hold everything together and go on. I didn't know exactly where we were heading, but I knew that I had to be strong for Jade, and I knew that I had to keep my emotions intact.

I carried Jade back to her room. With this dying child in my arms, I stood outside the doorway, looking in. There were other parents there visiting with their children. Everyone was laughing and having a good time. I couldn't stop myself from staring at this other world, a world of hope and happiness. They *should* laugh, I thought. Their child is going to get better. Their child is going home to live a long, happy, normal life. God, how unfair it is! Why did You exclude us from this kind of world?

Realizing that I was once again losing a grip on my emotions, I placed Jade in her bed, gave her the photo album to look at, and told her that I was going to the cafeteria to have supper.

Instead, I paced up and down the corridor of the cardiology ward, wondering where the hell I was going to get the strength to carry on.

As I lay awake on the playroom cot that night, all I could think about was getting Jade away from this dreadful place. She needed to be at home, and I needed to be strong for her. "God," I prayed, "You seem to ignore my every prayer, but if You have a heart at all, You'll give me strength. It's the very least You can do for us now, in this desperate time of need."

It occurred to me that I hadn't even asked the doctor how long Jade was expected to live. Maybe he told me, but maybe I didn't hear him. I started to cry again. "Prepare myself." Oh, Jesus, it hurt so much!

I then resolved that I didn't want to know Jade's life expectancy. Knowing, I thought, would just hurt all the more. I also decided that I would reveal this painful news to as few people as necessary.

The next day, Saturday, I requested an afternoon pass from the hospital so that I could take Jade for an outing. She was absolutely thrilled when I told her that we were meeting Grandma for lunch at the nearby shopping plaza. There was also another special surprise in store for her: Santa Claus and a Christmas puppet show.

Jade enjoyed going to restaurants. "I wuv it!" she exclaimed, as she started to eat her tuna salad. She also loved to see so many people again, the Christmas decorations, and the toy store where her grandmother bought her whatever toy her little heart desired.

After going down the escalator to the main floor, Jade excitedly leaped out of her stroller.

"Santa Cause!" she screamed. "Santa here, wookit, wookit!"

She stood in the lineup, then impatiently inched her way

to the front of the line. My mother and I were joyous as we watched this little angel, with her big, beautiful, happy smile, raising her arms to be lifted to Santa's lap.

Jade's picture was taken, and she was ecstatic when Santa handed her a couple of candy canes.

"Wookit, Gamma. Wookit, Mommy. Santa gimme canny canes."

She then scurried off, returning to the end of the line for a second visit. As I was about to go after her, my mother tugged at my sleeve, saying, "Leave her be, she's happy."

I couldn't get over it—the instant energy Jade managed to find when she first spotted Santa.

Returning Jade to her hospital bed wasn't easy. She cried, "Wanna go home, Mommy." I told her, "Tomorrow, Jade, I promise." And it was a promise I fully intended to keep, regardless of what the doctors might have had in mind.

The cardiologist agreed that it would be best to take Jade home. There were some changes made to her medication that seemed to help, and she hadn't experienced any chest pains during her four-day hospital stay.

At home, Jade remained in bed over the next few days. At her request, the television was brought into her bedroom so she could watch her favourite shows: *Mr. Rogers' Neighbourhood*, *Sesame Street*, *Polka Dot Door*, and *The Littlest Hobo*. Many times throughout the day, I brought in a tray of food. Jade nibbled a little, then asked that the tray be removed.

Jade was interested in books again, especially the stories about Jesus, but something itched deep inside me. I wanted somehow for Jade to be prepared for the day that we would no longer be together. I didn't quite know what to say or how to explain it, but it was so important to me that Jade receive some sort of honest explanation. More than anything I didn't want her to be frightened. *Death*. The word in itself frightened me, yet I didn't want Jade to be afraid.

I explained to her that Jesus loved her just as much as I did and, because He loved her so much, He would someday want her to come to live with Him. Sitting beside me on her bed, Jade was silent. She listened intently, absorbing every word.

"Jesus thinks you are very special and He would love to take care of you someday. Would you like to live with Jesus someday?"

Jade thought about my question but didn't answer.

"Jesus," I continued, "lives in Heaven—a beautiful world with lots of warm sunshine all the time. There are lots of beautiful trees and flowers. There are small animals that you can feed and take care of. There are lots of other children to play with and lots of toys. You can play all your favourite games."

"Duck-duck-goose?" she asked. "And tisket-tasket?"

"Oh yes, Jade. And baseball, too. Wouldn't that be great?"

Jade smiled a little but still never answered my question.

"So someday, Jade, would you like to live in Heaven with Jesus?"

"You too, Mommy? You coming, too?"

"Yes, Jade, I'll come too, but maybe not right away. Maybe Jesus will want to spend some time with you alone first. But as soon as He wants me, I'll come right away, and we'll both live together in Heaven, and we'll be very happy. Maybe we should say a prayer to Jesus, reminding Him that we wish to be together."

Jade agreed. After I said a short prayer, she added, "God bess Mommy."

I left the room just as Jade fell asleep, then went to my own room to cry. Please, God, let everything I told Jade be the truth.

CHAPTER FIFTEEN

The change in Jade's medication seemed to work wonders. Her health appeared to be improving with each passing day. Her appetite was back to normal; she gained a few pounds; her colour was good; she was less fatigued, and she was in high spirits.

We started preparing for Christmas early this year, and Jade once again had a zest for life. She was energetic, eagerly helping to decorate the house and drawing pictures of Santas, reindeer, Christmas trees, and presents.

She was pleased when her kindergarten teacher came to the house to visit. Linda, the special-ed teacher, came as well, but to teach. "I want to do it," Linda assured me. "If Jade can't come to school, well, then we'll have to bring the school to Jade."

For about an hour each morning, Linda sat with Jade at the desk in Jade's bedroom, working with her each day, providing new and interesting activities.

One morning they wrote a letter to Santa. When Linda had left, Jade showed me the sealed envelope and requested that we send it right away. "Wetter for Santa," she said, "Quick, quick, put in mayo box."

That afternoon, just as Jade dropped the letter into the mailbox, a postman arrived to collect the contents from the box. Jade started to worry. "No, no," she said in a panic, "Put back wetter. Wetter fer Santa, no you!"

The postman walked off, and I walked home with this crying child, trying to explain how our government's postal system works.

At least twice a day over the next week, Jade checked our

mailbox. With a look of disappointment on her face, she walked slowly up the stairs, saying, "No wetter foe Jade. Aah."

I was about to write the letter myself, forging Santa's signature, when finally it arrived. Jade was ecstatic. "Wookit, Mommy, wookit. Santa gimme wetter!"

I attempted to read the typewritten form letter when Jade yanked it from my hand, then pointed to *her* name that was printed on it. As I walked away, she started to apologize, "I sowee Gayo, you weed it."

The letter was then placed in her pink tote bag, never to leave her sight.

Jade appeared to have made a miraculous recovery. It was as though she had never been sick.

Two weeks before Christmas, I brought her to the hospital for her cardiology appointment. The ultrasound showed a loss of fluid, which of course was good. The doctors were amazed.

"I'm so impressed," Dr. Gibbons had said. "I haven't seen Jade looking so healthy in a long time. Her colour is good, her heart sounds good, and I see she's put on some weight. I'm happy to tell you that Jade seems to have finally beaten that virus. That's wonderful! In no time at all, she'll probably be better than she's ever been."

Happy, wonderful, beautiful thoughts raced through my mind. I must have had a grin from ear to ear. "Jade has fooled us all. She *is* better than she's ever been!"

After the appointment, my mother met Jade and me at McDonald's. Although I disliked fast food places, it was Jade's choice, and anything she wanted now was absolutely fine with me.

She placed her own order: a milkshake and animal crackers. She devoured the entire so-called meal. We then went to see a movie at the cinema in the nearby shopping plaza.

Jade didn't pay much attention to the comedy, *The Peanut Butter Solution*. Instead she observed the people around her, laughing when they laughed, and commenting, "Funny movie, eh, Gamma? Funny movie, eh, Mommy?"

When the film was over, Jade didn't walk, but *ran* out of the cinema, laughing hysterically. Onlookers couldn't help but to stop, look, and laugh. I simply couldn't believe my eyes. In the past, Jade had never been able to run so quickly. She dashed out into the plaza with a loud squeal of delight.

"Santa Cause!" she screamed. "Here *gen*!"

Sure enough the jolly old fellow was seated at the centre of the mall, while parents had their wallets handy to pay for their children's grand photo session.

My mother and I could hardly keep up with Jade. She didn't inch her way to the front of the lineup. Instead, she jumped the queue, politely telling the other children, "Move it, pease."

Standing by, watching Jade as she sat on Santa's lap, I was the happiest person in the world—so happy that I wanted to scream out and cheer, but managed to contain myself. I looked at my mother. "All I can say, Ma, is this has got to be a miracle—a real miracle!"

There were a lot of smiling, happy faces when Jade returned to school. Life, finally, was back to normal again, and I was "preparing myself." I was preparing myself for a fulfilling, meaningful, happy future with my precious, precious daughter.

Andrew came by one morning and surprised Jade with a Christmas tree. "This is for you," he said, "and after it's all decorated, Santa is going to put lots of presents under it on Christmas morning."

I then asked Jade, "How would you like Emmanuel to come over to help decorate the tree?"

Jade was overjoyed. "All wite! Mammo come helping me!"

After hanging a few decorations, Jade and Emmanuel headed to the bedroom where they found better things to do, such as playing floor hockey. Joan and I, though not unwillingly, finished decorating the tree while enjoying the sounds of laughter coming from the other room.

Jade attended several Christmas parties, and later she joyfully announced, "I love it. I love Kissmas. I love you. I love Santa. I love Joan and Jim. I love Gamma and Poppa. I love fends. And I love evabody!"

"And everybody loves you, too, Jade!"

It was another wonderful Christmas. After mass, Andrew, Jade, and I went over to my parents' house for the traditional turkey dinner. Jade opened some gifts, and my father, much to my surprise, offered to dress up as this year's Santa.

Jade sat on Santa's knee, looking at him very suspiciously. There really was no mistaking his voice. After a few minutes of uncertainty, Jade decided that he *must* be Santa, and she started to tell him what she had for supper that night.

When Santa supposedly left the house, Jade returned to the kitchen to play with the live gifts Andrew and I gave her a couple of weeks before Christmas. Two ferrets, named Fred and Farah, went scurrying about the house while Jade tried to catch them.

(After reading and hearing about the therapeutic use of animals as a way of raising the morale of the sick, elderly, or handicapped, I had decided that despite my allergies, it was definitely worth a try. Jade had the responsibility of feeding Fred and Farah twice daily, as well as the responsibility of helping to bathe them once a week.)

A few days after Christmas, Jade came down with a seemingly mild cold. But she may have also been experiencing, as many of us do, the Christmas letdown. All the weeks of preparation, the excitement and anticipation of Christmas day, the Christmas parties—and now it was all over. Christmas had passed.

Concerned about Jade's morale, Andrew and I planned a few activities. Because Jade enjoyed going for car drives, Andrew made a point of taking her out for a drive each morning. She enjoyed listening to the car radio as she quietly sang along. Her voice grew louder when a familiar song came on, one she knew almost all the words to: Boy George's, *Karma Chameleon.*

Later in the morning we brought her out on her sled, then

built three snowmen, one for each of us. After lunch, Jade took a long nap, then played with some of her new toys for a while.

In the evening, we sat by the fireplace in Andrew's spacious, but cosy living room. Jade sat beside Andrew on the sofa and was quite content as she listened to the soft notes he was strumming on his guitar. She then started to strum a few notes herself, inventing her own songs to sing. The energy wasn't there though, not as it had been at Christmastime.

Within a few more days, Jade's cold had become congested, and her appetite was rapidly decreasing. She became more and more fatigued, sleeping for longer periods at a time.

On an almost daily basis, I had been in touch with the cardiology nurse and kept her informed of Jade's state of health. She advised, "Due to Jade's recent illness, and the further deterioration of her heart, it can be expected that she would not be able to combat a common cold as well as she had in the past." She added, "I've relayed this information to Dr. Gibbons, and he suggests that you treat the cold as you always have and ensure that Jade gets plenty of fluids and rest."

Over the next few days, Jade became extremely listless. She was now sleeping twenty hours per day. She could no longer sleep in a horizontal position, and one night, the chest pains recurred. She woke up screaming, "Tummy hutts, Mommy, tummy hutts!"

I leaped out of bed and rushed to her room. Jade was sitting up in bed with a terrified look on her face. Her arms were folded around her stomach as she cried, "Bad dweam, Mommy. Had bad dweam."

I tried to comfort her. "Oh poor Jade, you had a bad dream? What did you dream about?"

She shrugged her shoulders, replying, "Don't know, Mommy, don't know." Then the tears started. "Stay wif me, I cared."

"Don't be afraid," I said. "Sometimes I have bad dreams too, but that's all they are, just dreams. Don't be scared." I then asked, "Jade, why are you holding your stomach? Does it hurt?"

She shook her head, saying, "Tummy hurts. Had bad

dweam."

I held her in my arms, rocking her for the rest of the night.

Early the next morning, I called the hospital and spoke with yet another new resident cardiologist. I was so broken up that I could barely get the words out. "It's starting all over again," I cried. The chest pains. They're happening again!"

The doctor advised me to bring Jade in for an examination. As I dressed her in her snowsuit, she pleaded, "No checkup, Mommy! Please no more checkup!"

Within an hour, my former roommate, Jennifer, picked us up and drove us to the hospital. After the examination was completed, this new doctor to Jade's case said, "It's just a cold, and because of Jade's recent illness, we have to expect that it's going to take longer for her to fight it." She added, "Jade isn't too congested and her heart sounds good; try not to worry so much."

I simply couldn't accept this, though. How could she possibly know that Jade was going to be all right? She was new to Jade's case, so how could she possibly know? I told her, "I don't think what Jade has is just a cold. What about the chest pains? Last night Jade woke up, crying that her stomach was hurting."

"Well, maybe it was just that," the doctor replied. "Maybe it was just a stomach ache. Her heart sounds good and, as I mentioned, her chest isn't too congested."

"No, it's more than a cold," I persisted. "Jade had once been diagnosed as having a touch of bronchitis, but what she actually had was a severe case of pneumonia—and heart failure."

I couldn't stop there as there was just too much to say. "Then there was the time when she was admitted to the hospital for several days and ended up there for several weeks. And then there was the time when the fluid around her heart was supposed to be removed, but it all came back." At this point, I was nearly hysterical. "I know everybody here is doing their best, but I also know from experience that sometimes the doctors are incorrect in their diagnoses. Listen," I explained, "I need Jade's regular cardiologist to examine her, and if he agrees with your diagnosis,

163

then I will accept it."

"I don't know if Dr. Gibbons is here right now," she said. "He was here all night performing an emergency surgery."

"Well," I said, "I'm not leaving until Dr. Gibbons examines Jade personally. I'm sorry, but you can't even *imagine* the hell that we've been going through!"

Within the hour Dr. Gibbons came in to see Jade. After the examination, he confirmed what the other doctor had told me. Just a cold.

Over the next few days, Jade showed no signs of improvement—none whatsoever. Off and on during the day and night, she fell into a deep sleep, but thankfully, she hadn't been experiencing any chest pains. Throughout the day there was soft music playing, all of Jade's favourite Raffi records.

Every few hours, in order to give Jade a change of scenery, I carried her to another room. I lay in my double bed with her for a while and read some of her favourite stories. I propped up some pillows on the living room sofa while Jade watched television, and occasionally, I brought her to our downstairs neighbour's house for a short visit. I was ready to do anything to comfort her and spark some interest—interest in anything but sleep. In order that we could keep each other company while I was washing dishes or preparing meals, I sat Jade's frail little body on a cushion on the kitchen floor, her back supported against the wall. Jade showed some interest in these minor changes during the day, but only for a short time. What she preferred was being held in my arms, having me stroke her hair and her face.

One morning, while I was holding a cup of juice for Jade to drink from, I noticed small white patches on her tongue. It's thrush, I thought. She's had it before. I telephoned the cardiology nurse and informed her of this discovery. "Thank goodness," she said. "Thrush is something we *can* treat, and it's probably the cause of Jade's loss of appetite and energy. It won't be necessary to bring her to the hospital. Simply bring her to your pediatrician for a prescription." She added, "Once the thrush has been treated, Jade will regain her appetite and build up the strength she needs in order to fight her cold."

After obtaining the prescription, I asked Joan to care for Jade that weekend so I could take a much-needed break. Jade was pleased with this plan, for she had always loved to spend time with Jim, Joan, and Emmanuel.

As I was preparing Jade's weekend bag, she was sitting on the living room sofa. Dressed in a new, pretty jogging suit, she sat up straight, legs crossed, trying to look alert, but she had to fight to keep her eyes open. I then sat beside her, showing her the photos that were taken at Christmastime. She stared at each photo with complete concentration for a minute or two, then placed each one back in the envelope.

She managed a smile and a brief giggle as she stared at one particular picture. It was the photo of her sitting on Santa's lap. She pointed to the red suit, admitting something that she must have known all along: "Poppa's in dare." I couldn't stop laughing. Why she never let on before, I don't know, but maybe, just maybe, she didn't want to ruin the fun for anyone else.

When leaving the house, I lifted Jade to carry her down the stairs. "Cawfoe wif me, Mommy, cawfoe." Through her illness, Jade had become so frail that even the slightest exertion was painful.

I placed her in her stroller and walked the few blocks to Joan's house. During our walk, I told Jade that I would be spending the weekend at Andrew's and that I would return for her on Sunday.

Although at first Jade was pleased at the idea of spending the weekend at Joan's, suddenly she was unsure. When we were halfway there, she said, "Wanna go home now, Mommy."

"But, Jade," I said, "I thought you wanted to visit Jim and Joan for a while."

She gave it some thought. Then, still with a bit of uncertainty, she very hesitantly said, "Okay."

After giving Joan fully detailed instructions concerning medication, I kissed Jade good-bye. "I love you, Jade. See you on Sunday."

As I was walking back home, where I was to meet Andrew

in a couple of hours, I had this awful, gnawing feeling of insecurity. I couldn't stop thinking about Jade. She seemed so uncertain all of a sudden about leaving me this weekend. I contemplated cancelling my weekend plans and returning for her. Over the next hour, I packed my weekend bag, unpacked, then repacked. I finally resolved, perhaps out of selfishness, that I needed the break and that Jade needed the change of scenery.

I didn't sleep well that night and Joan called the next morning.

"Jade has been awake coughing most of the night," Joan said. "We placed her on the living room couch this morning, and she's been dozing off and on. Jim and I are taking turns sitting with her. She seems to be more comfortable when someone is with her at all times. I've been giving Jade her medicine right on schedule, and this afternoon, after a good rest, maybe she'll enjoy a little outing in her stroller."

"Yes," I agreed, "the fresh air will do her some good."

That afternoon I said to Andrew, "This is crazy. I'm not getting a break. I just can't stop worrying. All I can do is hope and pray that the treatment for Jade's thrush will start taking effect."

"Listen, Gail, if you want, we can drive to Joan's right now and bring Jade to your house. Maybe you'll worry less if you were with her."

I thought about it a while, then decided, "No, Jade is in excellent care. I trust Joan totally, and she'll call me if anything comes up. I'm just as worried about myself right now. I'm worried that if I don't take my mind off Jade for a while, emotionally, I won't be giving her my best while she's recovering. I need to put my thoughts elsewhere for a while. Let's go for a hike in the woods tomorrow; then, later in the day, as planned, we'll pick up Jade."

I would soon find out that if ever I was going to make a poor judgement call, this was it.

The next morning, January 12, Joan called me. "Gail, I hate to worry you, but we're really concerned about Jade. She hardly slept at all last night. She had difficulty breathing and was coughing incessantly. With a pillow and some blankets, she spent the night in the bathroom. I thought the steam from the running shower would help. And this morning she absolutely refused to take her medication. Jim and I think we should bring her to the hospital."

I started to cry. "No, wait," I said, "I'll call the hospital first and arrange for Jade to be admitted. I want to avoid her having to be examined by the emergency staff."

It was all arranged. That afternoon Jade was to be admitted to the cardiology ward for tests, and I would meet Joan at the hospital.

Joan arrived at the hospital early and called me right away. "Don't rush, Gail. Jade is fine, and I'm with her. She doesn't seem worried in the least; she's just sitting up in bed now, looking around. She hasn't put up any fuss, and she knows that you're coming."

Relieved, I said, "Fine. Before going to the hospital then, I'll go home to get some of Jade's things. I'm sure she'll want some of her dolls and books."

As we pulled up at the hospital, I said to Andrew, "Listen, I would like to spend some time with Jade alone for a while, so if you have other things to do, please feel free to do them. I'm sure that we're going to be here all night, so you can come back later if you want."

As I headed down the corridor of the cardiology ward, I instantly sensed that something was wrong. A nurse ran over to me, took me by the arm and led me to the nurses' lounge, which was located just opposite Jade's room. As we were walking, I kept turning my head toward the room. There were many doctors and nurses surrounding one of the beds.

As we entered the lounge, I noticed Joan sitting on the sofa, a look of despair on her face.

The nurse put both her hands on my shoulders, and my body went limp. "What happened?" I cried.

"Jade went into cardiac arrest," she said.

"Oh no, my poor baby!"

"The doctors are doing everything they can to revive her,

and I think it's best if you stay here in this room in the meantime."

I sat next to Joan on the sofa. "What happened?" I asked.

"Jade seemed to be fine," she explained, "She was sitting on the bed, watching everything that was going on around her, when suddenly she doubled over. I thought she had fainted, and I immediately picked her up and called out for a doctor. Within a minute, doctors and nurses came rushing in and—Gail, they're doing everything they can."

"When did this happen?" I asked.

"It happened about fifteen minutes before you arrived."

I jumped up when one of the doctors entered the room. It was the same doctor who had examined Jade about a week ago. "Is she okay?" I asked. Is she okay now?"

"Gail, the doctors are doing everything they can. They got Jade's heart beating for about a minute, but it stopped again. I think she's going to die."

"I need to hold her," I cried. "Please, I need to hold her!"

"You can see her if you like, Gail," the doctor said. "But it would probably be easier for everyone if you'd just let the doctors work. They are still trying to revive Jade, and it isn't a pleasant sight."

I stood by the door of the lounge and looked through the window at the room across the hall. Then, pacing the floor of the small lounge, I pleaded, "Let her be okay, God. Please, let her be okay."

A few minutes later, the doctor re-entered the room. There were tears in her eyes. She put her hand on my shoulder and said, "Jade died."

"What? She's okay?" I asked.

"No," the doctor said as she placed a firmer grip on my shoulder. "Gail, I said she died. It was her time."

I sat down and cried until there were no more tears left to shed. There was a cold dread in my heart. I wanted to hate God, but for Jade's sake, I wanted to love Him now more than ever. I wanted to thank Him for ending Jade's suffering, but at the same time, I wasn't sure if this gratitude was justified.

The doctor sat beside me and informed me that the nurses were now washing Jade, and that I could see her in a short while. Joan tried to comfort me. "You did your best for Jade," she said. "You gave her everything. You both loved each other so much, and Jade had a good life. She's no longer suffering. She's in good hands now."

One of the nurses entered the lounge. "You can see Jade now if you wish."

I looked at this beautiful, precious, little girl who was so peaceful now and no longer experiencing any pain. My own pain seemed to be subsiding a little as I looked at Jade. Her eyes were wide open, staring into the nothingness of this world. She's gone, I thought. Her body is here, but she's gone.

I leaned over the bed to hold her and kiss her beautiful face. "Jade," I cried, "I'm here, my precious, and I love you so much. Remember Jesus? Well, He's going to take care of you from now on. I love you, Jade. Please hear me. I love you so much."

Joan and I returned to the lounge where we were joined by a cardiology doctor and the intensive care doctor. One doctor said to me, "It was as though Jade knew. Somehow, I think that even small children can sense when death is near. When Joan brought Jade to the hospital, Jade seemed to be relieved. She didn't even try to put up a fight, and much to my amazement, she spoke so clearly right until the end."

She continued, "Jade was in a complete state of resignation. When I was taking a blood sample from her, she whimpered, then said, 'That's all now. No more.' It was her time. Her heart was just too tired to function any more."

Jim arrived at the hospital. "How's Jade," he asked.

"Jimmy, Jade is dead," Joan replied.

They both went into the room to see Jade.

The doctors sat with me, then broached the subject of an autopsy. "Normally," they said, "if a child dies after being in the

169

hospital's care for less than twenty-four hours, an autopsy is legally required. But in Jade's case, we know the cause. In any event, however, you may wish to know the exact details of the cause of death. Although you may not feel that way right now, you may have questions sometime in the future. Also, autopsies are very educational for the doctors, helping them to acquire more knowledge concerning diseases and so forth."

Without any hesitation, I replied, "No. No autopsy. Throughout Jade's life, she had been subjected to so many tests, but no more. I don't want anyone to touch her any more. Just leave her be in peace. Jade is gone now, and that's information enough for me."

And it was left at that.

CHAPTER SIXTEEN

The funeral was held on January 15, 1986, at two o'clock in the afternoon, an occasion that remains mostly a blur. About the only thing I could remember with any amount of clarity was the eulogy:

> Jade, I want you to know,
> You have given us something special
> That we all can cherish so dear:
> Your love, your humour, and sweetness,
> And in our hearts you'll always be here.
>
> You had the ability to reach out to others –
> You did it, darling, just with a smile.
> Your innocence and affection
> And your limits knew no mile.
>
> Your delightful ways touched people's lives,
> Because you've always had the will
> To do your best in everything,
> Which was your greatest skill.
>
> And we have to believe, my precious,
> That you've lived a very full life,
> Always so happy and busy and eager,
> From early morning 'til night.

Remember baby Jesus?
We talked about Him a lot.
He wants you home with Him now,
And He's so proud of all you've taught.

Can't imagine life without you, though –
It hurts to even try,
But I know Jesus will keep you warm
And always walk by your side.

And please remember, my darling,
That a part of you is with me,
A bond which cannot be broken –
And, I promise, it'll never be.

After the funeral, after the reception, after everything was over, I spent the night at my parents' house. I returned home the following day. I didn't want anyone around me, not even Andrew—especially not Andrew. I was still trying to deal with the guilt feelings of having been with him—instead of Jade—when she died.

Unable to bring myself to leave Jade's bedroom, I felt sad and empty. I was inundated with cards and letters. I was especially moved by a letter written by Jade's former foster father, which read in part:

Dear Gail,

I have been surprised by the deep impact Jade's death has had on me. Her problem was predicted from a very young age, and Jade was seriously sick for the second time since October, neither eating nor sleeping properly. The last trip to the hospital was confirmation of the seriousness. But Joan's words, 'Jade is dead,' really hit hard.

In a way, seeing Jade lying so peaceful, so beautiful in death on her hospital bed, was a relief. She had found a haven from her suffering, from her struggle to breathe, from her inability to eat and sleep, from a world that had dealt her a tough hand. Jade's death seems to be occupying my thoughts much more than I would have imagined.

Ironic, isn't it? Down syndrome with congenital heart defect, requiring (and demanding, as only she could) lots of care and attention. By many of society's standards, she would not—could not—even come close to succeeding in life. Yet who more than Jade succeeded in eliciting genuine, deep emotion from everybody who passed her way even briefly? She truly touched a lot of people. She had a way of capturing hearts.

Jade had an ability to attract. I know of no one who was unmoved by her lovable simplicity. And she has inspired feelings of true altruism—in our whole family, most assuredly in me.

Jade was a person of great importance to all of us.

Thank you for sharing Jade with us. She brought a real joy to our lives. But our happiness was not because of Jade alone: it was the story of Jade and Gail. Our job as foster parents came to the most satisfactory completion when Jade returned to your care. We laughingly called ourselves foster grandparents after that, and were quite comfortable with the title, and very pleased that we could get to spoil Jade for the occasional weekend.

Because of you, we enjoyed a very special person in Jade. Because of Jade, you are very special to us.

I heard you pray at Jade's wake, asking God to take care of your baby whom you are going to miss so. How much more clearly God hears such a genuine appeal!

She was sent to us by God as a messenger of love. He saw that she had done her job well, and called her back to Him to receive her eternal reward. She is safe now, well taken care of; she is far better off than we.

I think I have learned to accept things that cannot be changed, and one of them is that a very good person has been taken away from us, and the world must continue.

But think how privileged, enriched, and blessed we are that Jade passed our way.

I wish I had the magic to make all your pain disappear, but I know that's impossible.

Maybe, just maybe, what I have written will bring you some small consolation; that has been my purpose. These words are meant to convey our love and support for you.

Jim

Over the next week, I spent a lot of time reading and rereading letters and cards of sympathy, trying to find as much comfort as I could. But I still couldn't manage to absorb it all—I had moments when virtual disbelief mingled with anger and denial. Did it really happen? Did Jade really die? God, why did she have to die? And why was I still praying for a miracle?

As I sat in Jade's bedroom, I was remembering all of the warmth and love that had filled this very room. Jade's drawings and paintings were still hanging on the walls, her cars and trucks still lying on the floor; the lonely doll house, with all the tiny figurines gathered around, sat as she had left it, and the colourful tote bags, which once carried many of Jade's prized possessions, had now been abandoned.

I looked at Jade's wooden desk and thought about the many wonderful hours we had sat there doing puzzles, reading stories, drawing pictures, and playing card games.

I felt Jade's presence. She was still here. But oh God, how I wish she *was* still here!

I was lying in Jade's bed, trying to feel her warmth, when I noticed Jo-Jo propped up against a cushion at the foot of the bed. With a big painted smile on her face, she stared at me, the band-aids still adhering to her arms and legs. She was Jade's favourite doll, and I held her tightly. I prayed again for a miracle—maybe the doll could be transformed into Jade. Please, God, bring her back to me. I need her . . .

My thoughts flashed back to the Christmas holidays. I

174

remembered all the fun we'd had. I thought of Jade's happy face, excited as she always had been about Christmas festivities. I started to laugh. Then I thought about the hospital, with all of its painful memories, and I started to cry.

What about the funeral? Did it actually take place? Was that really my little girl in that small white casket? I remember talking to her. Did she hear me?

I was no longer afraid of death—not if it meant being reunited with Jade. Quite possibly, Jesus had answered one prayer. I had asked Him, on numerous occasions, to heal Jade. Maybe now she was healed.

I also remembered other prayers and tried to determine whether they'd been answered in any way at all. I remembered praying to Jesus that if it really wasn't His will to leave Jade with me, that He please not let her suffer. But she had suffered so much in the past few months. And now I was trying to be thankful that she had not suffered any longer. I wondered why children have to suffer at all, for they are so pure and innocent and free of sin.

Jade and I were a team. The deepest and most profound love and joy we shared was through each other. She had gone to be surrounded by Jesus' love, and I had to figure out a way to accept that.

It has been seventeen years since Jade died, but oftentimes I sense that her spirit is still with me.

It could be a smell I detect in a specialty shop we had both visited, or it could be the scent of a body lotion, or it could be a song that we both enjoyed listening to, or a familiar-sounding giggle, or a silly situation when I've felt that I've been there before. It could be a dream, mostly a happy one, though always the endings are sad. Out of nowhere, I might still hear some of Jade's funny sayings and remember various humorous situations. And sadly, I still feel pangs of guilt that I just can't seem to shake, at least not until I envision Jade's ever-forgiving face.

I'm not angry any more. I hold no hostility toward anyone, not even toward God, as we have an agreement to which I fully intend to hold Him.

There is no one else in this world who can replace Jade, or replace the love that we shared, but I've since learned that there is other love.

Andrew and I married five months after Jade died. We have three wonderful, healthy children: a daughter, Lindsay, now aged sixteen; a son, Mark, aged fourteen; and another son, Stephen, aged nine.

In 1997, we moved to Victoria, British Columbia. Andrew and I anticipated the day that we could make this major life change and start something new in fresh surroundings—add more adventure to our lives. And that we did. Now living in the midst of lush forests, hiking trails, lakes, mountains, and wildlife, we certainly have found adventure.

I still have dreams of Jade, though they're getting scarcer and scarcer. This worries me, for I never, ever, wish to be left with only photographs and memories. But if dreams are perhaps impermanent, Jade's love is ever-present, for I could not have written this story without her spirit sitting alongside me—helping me to remember her—through every emotionally charged minute.

I still have bouts of extreme sadness. Yet these are also the times when a small, precious angel looks down on me and, in her most sympathetic voice, comforts me with her own special wisdom.

"Aah, no sad, Mommy, kay?"

ACKNOWLEDGEMENTS

I could not have written this book without the help of others, namely, my husband and best friend, Andrew McInnes, whose loving support and wholehearted encouragement saw me through even the most trying moments, when I had all but given up. I am grateful to my children, Lindsay, Mark and Stephen. They allowed me this time to write, often fending for themselves, tidying the house, preparing meals, and understanding that my "silent treatments" were not directed at them, but were merely moments of reflection as I completed each chapter.

A special thanks to my wonderful editor and literary consultant, Patricia Anderson, for her ongoing support and mentoring.

I am grateful to Jim and Joan Pearson for taking the time to read my rough draft and gently teach me about a few grammatical rules.

A big *thank you* to my dearest friend, Johanna Deheer, for her invaluable time and patience in helping me with the final touch-ups.

My thanks also to award-winning cover illustrator, Sheena Lott, who was already over-committed with work, yet made an exception for Jade's story.

My deepest gratitude goes to my little angel. In the closing of Jade's memoir, I wrote, "… Jade's love is ever-present, for I could not have written this story without her spirit sitting alongside me—helping me to remember her—through every emotional minute." And you know what? That's the God's honest truth, since I have no other explanation for how I remembered all the details of our life together.

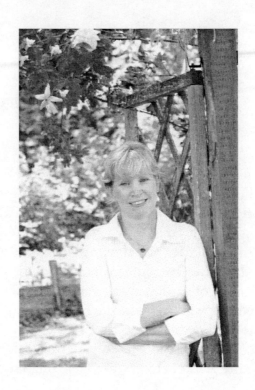

ABOUT THE AUTHOR

I grew up in Montréal, Quebéc, the fourth of eight children. I am married and have three wonderful children. Having earlier had a child with Down syndrome and a congenital heart defect, I long felt the need to convey the spirit and meaning of my daughter Jade's brief life.

In writing *Natural Harmony*, my intention was to move, to inspire, and to educate people about the injustices dealt to those born with distinct challenges. As well, I wanted to share some of the joy that I found in the love and laughter of my sweet little girl.

ISBN 141200392-X
9 781412 003926